사람마다 추구하는 꿈이 다르고 목표가 다르기 때문에, 각자의 인생 경로는 다양하고 독특합니다. 어떤 사람은 학문적 성취를 꿈꾸며 연구와 공부에 몰두하고, 또 어떤 사람은 창의적인 예술 활동을 통해 자신의 열정을 표현합니다. 또한, 누군가는 안정적인 직업과 가족을 이루는 것을 목표로 하기도 합니다. 이와 같은 개인의 다양한 목표와 꿈은 삶의 다양성을 보여주며, 우리의 사회를 더욱 풍요롭게 만듭니다.

인생의 여정에서 새로운 도전을 시작하는 것은 때로는 두렵지만, 그만큼 가치 있는 일입니다. 특히 간호사라는 전문직을 가지고 새로운 나라에서 경력을 이어가고자 하는 결정은 큰 용기가 필요한 선택일 것입니다.

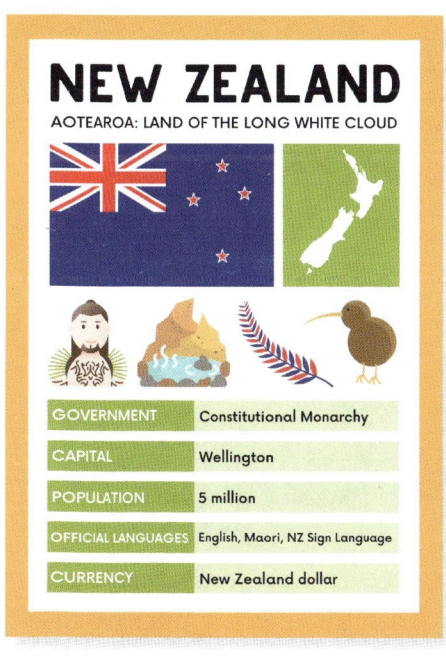

_____ 님께

_____ 드림

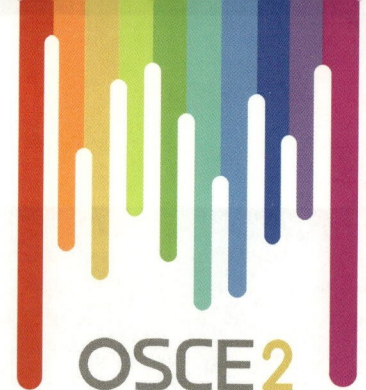

OSCE2
국제간호사를 위한 **임상술기시험**

첫째판 1쇄 인쇄 | 2025년 4월 5일
　　　1쇄 발행 | 2025년 4월 10일

저　　자 | 김라경
발 행 인 | 모형중
편 집 인 | 모형중
디 자 인 | 이명호

발 행 처 | 포널스
등　　록 | 제2017-000021호
본　　사 | 서울시 강북구 노해로8길22 경남아너스 3층
창　　고 | 서울시 강북구 노해로8길22 경남아너스 2층
전　　화 | 02-905-9671　Fax | 02-905-9670

ⓒFORNURSE 2025년, 국제간호사를 위한 임상술기시험 OSCE Vol.2
Copyright©2025 ALL RIGHTS RESERVED

본서는 지은이와의 계약에 의해 포널스 출판사에서 발행합니다.
본서의 내용 및 삽화 일부 혹은 전부를 무단으로 전재 및 복제하는 것은 법으로 엄격히 금지되어 있습니다.

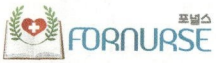
www.fornursebook.com

📖 도서 반품과 파본 교환은 본사로 문의하시기 바랍니다.
📖 검인은 저자와의 합의로 생략합니다.

ISBN　979-11-6627-641-5　93510
정　가　25,000원

국제간호사를 위한
임상술기시험
OSCE VOLUME 2

Objective Structured Clinical Examinations
객관적 구조와 임상 시험

김라경 지음

FORNURSE

뉴질랜드는 깨끗한 자연환경과 높은 삶의 질, 그리고 전문직 종사자들을 위한 우수한 근무 환경으로 전 세계의 주목을 받고 있습니다. 특히 의료 분야에서는 체계적인 시스템과 전문성을 인정받는 환경이 마련되어 있어, 많은 한국 간호사들이 새로운 기회를 찾아 뉴질랜드로의 진출을 고려하고 있습니다.

　　To become a Nurse in New Zealand 전자책을 발간하고 뉴질랜드 간호사를 꿈꾸는 많은 선생님들과 1:1 강의를 진행한 지 2년이 되어갑니다. 이 과정에서 저는 다양한 경력과 열정을 가진 분들을 만나며 함께 성장할 수 있었습니다. 확신할 수 있는 것은, 뉴질랜드 간호사라는 목표는 분명 도달 가능한 꿈이라는 것입니다.

　　2024년 말부터 뉴질랜드 간호협회(Nursing Council of New Zealand, NCNZ)는 해외 간호사 등록 절차에 새로운 변화를 도입했습니다. 이 변경 사항은 국제적으로 자격을 갖춘 간호사(Internationally qualified nurses : IQN)들이 뉴질랜드에서 일하기 위한 절차를 단순화하고 보다 공정하고 일관된 평가를 제공하는 것을 목표로 합니다. 변경 사항에 대한 자세한 정보는 뉴질랜드 간호협회 웹사이트에서 확인할 수 있습니다.

김 라 경

Contents

Part I

*1*장 뉴질랜드 간호사의 모든 것   9

이 책이 당신에게 필요한 이유   10

해외간호사의 뉴질랜드 간호사 취업 현황에 대한 동향과 변화   13

뉴질랜드 간호사의 이점   15

뉴질랜드 간호사의 연봉   20

해외 간호사가 뉴질랜드 간호사가 되기 위한 조건   23

뉴질랜드 간호협회의 주요 변경 사항   27

---

*2장*은 무지개 색상으로 구분하여 OSCE 시험의 특징적인 10가지 스테이션을 부각시키고, 10개 스테이션별로 4개의 세부적인 시나리오를 담아, 보다 깊이 있는 이해를 돕고자 합니다.

Part II

2장 10단계 예문과 단계별 4개 연습 시나리오   35

❶ 정신 건강 사정 36

- 연습 Scenario 1: Sadness and hopelessness   46
- 연습 Scenario 2: Mood swings and erratic behaviour   51
- 연습 Scenario 3: hearing voices and paranoid thoughts   57
- 연습 Scenario 4: Flashbacks and nightmares   63

❷ 신체사정(활력징후 측정) 69

- 연습 Scenario 1: Abdominal pain and nausea   77
- 연습 Scenario 2: Headaches and dizziness   83
- 연습 Scenario 3: Joint pain and swelling   89
- 연습 Scenario 4: Sudden onset of right-sided weakness   95

❸ 세부 생리학적 사정 101

- 연습 Scenario 1: Ileus Symptoms Management for Post-Colectomy Patient   111
- 연습 Scenario 2: Increased Intracranial Pressure(ICP) Symptoms Post-Craniotomy Surgery   119
- 연습 Scenario 3: Hyponatremia(Na 113) Post-Total Knee Replacement   128
- 연습 Scenario 4: Sore Throat After Holiday – Lymph Node Assessment   135

❹ 전문석인 답변 143

- 연습 Scenario 1: Informed Consent   150
- 연습 Scenario 2: Ethical Dilemma in Patient Care   154
- 연습 Scenario 3: Professional Boundaries   159
- 연습 Scenario 4: Advocating for a Patient's Cultural Needs   163

❺ 응급상황 관리 169

- 연습 Scenario 1: Severe Asthma Attack   178
- 연습 Scenario 2: Hypoglycaemic Emergency   182
- 연습 Scenario 3: Acute Myocardial Infarction(Heart Attack)   186
- 연습 Scenario 4: Seizure management   191

Contents

❻ 임상 술기(상처드레싱 교환) 195

연습 Scenario 1: Nasogastric tube Insertion	205
연습 Scenario 2: Changing a Colostomy Bag	213
연습 Scenario 3: Monitoring Blood Glucose Levels(BGLs)	221
연습 Scenario 4: Central Venous Catheter Dressing Method	228

❼ 약물 투약 237

연습 Scenario 1: Transdermal Patch Application	242
연습 Scenario 2: Inhalation Medication Administration	246
연습 Scenario 3: Clexane Injection after Total Hip Replacement (THR) due to Clotting Factor Disorder	251
연습 Scenario 4: Insulin Doses Calculation and Administration (Long-Acting vs Short-Acting Insulin)	258

❽ 의사소통 및 팀워크 267

연습 Scenario 1: Patient Education	272
연습 Scenario 2: Conflict Resolution	277
연습 Scenario 3: Crisis Communication	281
연습 Scenario 4: Communicating with a Patient with Limited English Proficiency	285

❾ 간호계획 수립 289

연습 Scenario 1: Diabetes Management	295
연습 Scenario 2: Palliative Care Plan	300
연습 Scenario 3: Paediatric Asthma Care Plan	305
연습 Scenario 4: Managing Acute Confusion in an Elderly Patient	310

❿ 위급한 상태의 환자 관리 315

연습 Scenario 1: Acute Gastrointestinal Bleed	322
연습 Scenario 2: Atrial Fibrillation with Rapid Ventricular Response(RVR)	326
연습 Scenario 3: Fall in a Hospitalized Patient with Signs of Deterioration	330
연습 Scenario 4: Deteriorating Post-Angioplasty Patient	335

OSCE 준비 꿀팁!   341

Part I

1장

뉴질랜드 간호사의
모든 것

이 책이 당신에게 필요한 이유

🔖 현실적이고 생생한 경험을 담다.

이 책은 제가 한국에서 뉴질랜드로 건너와 겪은 실제 경험을 바탕으로 작성되었습니다. 단순한 이론서가 아닌, 제가 직접 겪은 과정과 시행착오를 통해 얻은 노하우를 생생하게 담아 현실적이고 실용적인 가이드를 제공합니다. 뉴질랜드 간호사라는 꿈을 이루기 위해 필요한 모든 단계를 경험한 저의 생생한 커리어 라이프 스토리는 여러분에게 믿음직한 로드맵이 될 것이라고 장담합니다.

🔖 전 과정을 아우르는 종합 가이드

이 책은 뉴질랜드 간호사가 되기 위한 등록 과정, 취업, 그리고 현지의 다른 문화에 대한 이해를 돕는 것은 물론, 각 단계에서 필요한 준비 사항과 실용적인 팁까지 함께 제공합니다.

🔖 최신 정보와 동향 반영

뉴질랜드 간호계의 변화는 빠르게 이루어지고 있습니다. 이 책은 뉴질랜드의 의료 시스템과 간호계의 최신 동향을 반영하여 뉴질랜드에서 간호사로의 꿈을 꾸는 분들께 변화하는 환경에 대비할 수 있도록 할 것입니다. 또한, 간호사로서 직무를 수행하는 데 필요한 정보와 트렌드를 이해하는 데 도움을 줄 것입니다.

🖋 실용적인 조언과 팁 제공

이 책은 저의 경험을 바탕으로, 뉴질랜드 간호사로서 근무를 시작할 때 필수적인 실무(practice), 관련 영어 회화, 실용적인 조언, 그리고 유용한 팁들을 제공합니다.

🖋 효과적인 영어 학습 전략 제시

국제적인 간호 환경에서 일하기 위해서는 무엇보다 영어 능력이 필수적입니다. 특히 뉴질랜드 간호사 자격을 준비하며 OSCE (Objective Structured Clinical Examination, 객관적 구조화 임상시험)에 응시할 때, 영어로 전문성을 표현하는 능력은 성공의 핵심입니다. 이 책은 OSCE 준비에 필요한 영어 표현과 학습 팁을 함께 제공합니다. 간호와 관련된 시뮬레이션 상황에서 자주 사용되는 표현을 익히고, 효율적으로 영어 실력을 키울 수 있도록 돕는 구체적인 가이드를 제공합니다.

🖋 실무 중심의 병원 영어 가이드

OSCE 시험과 실제 병원 근무에서 가장 큰 장벽 중 하나는 언어입니다. 이 책은 해외 간호사들이 뉴질랜드 병원 환경에서 직면할 수 있는 상황을 중심으로 병원에서 실제로 사용되는 영어 표현과 의사소통 방법의 예를 정리했습니다. 환자와의 소통, 의료진과의 협력, 상황 보고 및 기록 작성 등 다양한 상황에 맞춘 실무 중심의 영어 가이드는 독자들이 OSCE 시험뿐만 아니라 실무에서도 자신감을 가질 수 있도록 도와줍니다.

한국에서 처음으로 발매되는 널싱 오스키 북, 이 책은 뉴질랜드 간호사 OSCE를 준비하는 모든 이들에게 실질적이고 체계적인 지침을 제공할것이라 믿습니다. 제가 직접 경험한 뉴질랜드 간호사 OSCE 준비 과정과 성공적인 시험 전략을 통해, 여러분에게 필요한 현실적 조언과 구체적인 실행 방안을 제시하고자 합니다.

이 책이 여러분에게 자신감을 불어넣고 뉴질랜드 간호사로서의 여정을 성공적으로 시작할 수 있도록 든든한 동반자가 되기를 바랍니다.

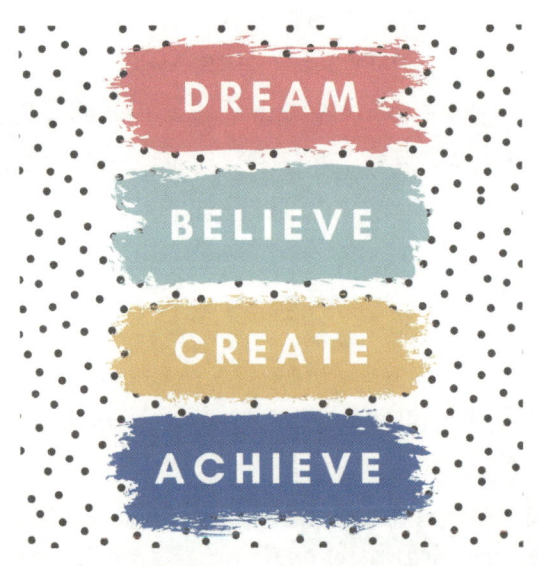

해외간호사의 뉴질랜드 간호사 취업 현황에 대한 동향과 변화

"뉴질랜드 간호사 취업 시장 동향"

📈 해외 간호사 유입 증가

코로나로 닫혔던 국경이 다시 열리게 되면서부터 해외 간호사들의 뉴질랜드 유입은 지속적으로 증가하는 추세입니다.

이전에는 CAP(Competence Assessment Programme) 코스를 이수해야 했지만, 2024년 말부터 도입된 뉴질랜드 간호협회의 새로운 시스템은 이론 시험과 OSCE(객관적 구조화 임상시험)를 통과하면 되는걸로 간략히 바뀌었습니다. 이로 인해 등록 비용도 크게 줄어든것고 더불어 시간도 절약되어 더 많은 해외 간호사들이 뉴질랜드 취업을 고려하고 있습니다.

📈 취업 기회의 변동

최근 해외 간호사들의 증가와 졸업생 수의 증가로 인해 취업 기회가 줄어들었다는 우려가 있습니다. 그러나 이는 개인의 상황에 따라 다를 수 있습니다. 개개인의 경력과 영어실력에 따라 다른 취업시장이니 정확하지 않은 뉴스에 너무 걱정할 필요는 없습니다. 또한 졸업생들이 취업의 기회를 얻지 못하는 이유에 대해서는 대부분의 보건 기관들이 경험 있는 간호사를 선호하기 때문입니다.

미래 인력 부족 우려

뉴질랜드 간호사 협회는 2035년까지 수요를 충족시킬 만큼의 충분한 간호사를 확보하지 못할 수 있다고 우려하고 있습니다. 이는 장기적으로 간호사 수요가 지속적으로 증가할 것임을 시사합니다.

결론적으로, 뉴질랜드 간호사가 되기 위한 간호협회의 시스템이 바뀌고 취업 시장이 변화하고 있지만, 해외 간호사들의 유입은 지속적으로 증가하고 있습니다. 장기적으로는 간호사 수요가 지속적으로 증가할 것으로 예상되어, 노력과 준비를 통해 취업 기회를 얻을 수 있을 것으로 보입니다.

뉴질랜드 간호사의 이점

한국 간호사가 뉴질랜드로 이직해야 하는 이유에 대해 솔직하게 이야기해 보도록 하겠습니다.

한국과 뉴질랜드의 간호 환경은 하늘과 땅 차이라고 할 수 있을 정도로 다르니까, 현실적인 부분을 자세히 짚어볼께요.

1 워라밸(Work-Life Balance): 삶의 질이 다름

🇰🇷 한국:

- 살인적인 교대근무, 야간 근무 많음
- 환자 대비 간호사 수 부족 → 업무 과중
- 병원 내 태움, 상급자 스트레스
- 휴가 눈치 보임, 연차 못 씀
- 퇴근 후에도 업무 연장(서류 작업, 교육 등)

🇳🇿 뉴질랜드:

- 하루 8시간 근무 철저하게 보장 (초과 근무 거의 없음)
- 환자 대비 간호사 수 적정 수준 유지 → 덜 바쁨
- 직장 내 존중 문화, 위계질서 약함
- 휴가 자유롭게 사용 가능 (연 4주 휴가 법적으로 보장)
- 퇴근 후 업무 연락 없음 (근무 외 시간은 철저히 개인 시간)

한국에서 간호사는 일을 위해 사는 느낌, 뉴질랜드에서는 일과 삶의 균형이 보장됨.

2. 급여 차이: 적은 스트레스로 더 많이 법니다.

 한국:

- 신입 간호사 초봉:
  약 3,500만 원~4,500만 원(야간 포함, 수당 포함)
- 경력 5년 차: 약 5,000만 원~6,000만 원
- 그러나 야근, 추가 근무, 위험 부담 감안하면 실질적 시급은 낮음

 뉴질랜드:

- 신입 간호사(Registered Nurse) 초봉:
  약 NZD 65,000~ 75,000 (한화 약 5,500만 원~6,500만 원)
- 경력 5년 차:
  NZD 85,000- 95,000 (한화 약 7,500만 원~8,500만 원)
- 야근 수당 별도, 추가 근무 거의 없음, 오버타임시 시급 2배 보장
- 세금 떼고도 실수령액이 한국보다 높음

한국보다 스트레스 적게 받고도 더 많이 번다.

3 직업 안정성 및 복지: 간호사 대우가 다름

 한국:

- 공공병원 적고 사립병원 많아, 병원 사정에 따라 근무 환경 크게 달라짐
- 산재 인정 어려움, 환자나 보호자의 폭언·폭행 빈번
- 육아휴직 쓰기 어려움

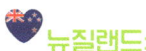 **뉴질랜드:**

- 간호사 노동조합(Union)이 강해서 근무 조건, 급여 협상 철저
- 병원에서 간호사를 함부로 대하지 않음 (노조가 강하게 보호)
- 환자가 간호사에게 폭언·폭행 시 바로 법적 조치
- 출산·육아휴직 자유롭고, 복직도 수월
- 정부 병원이 많아 직업 안정성이 높음

 뉴질랜드 간호사는 전문직으로 존중받으며, 노동권이 강하게 보호됨.

WORK / LIFE BALANCE

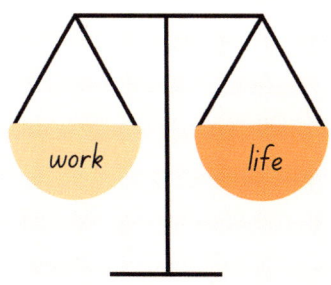

4 정신적·육체적 스트레스 차이

한국:

- 의료진이 부족해 한 명당 담당해야 하는 환자가 많음 → 초과 근무와 극심한 스트레스
- 태움, 꼰대 등으로 이루어진 특이한 상하관계로 인해 신규 간호사 퇴사율 높음
- 보호자 및 환자 컴플레인 심함
- 의료 사고 시 간호사가 법적 책임을 져야 하는 경우 많음

뉴질랜드:

- 환자 수가 적당해 간호사가 과로하지 않음 (보통 8시간 근무에 일반병동은 한명의 간호사가 환자 4명 돌봄)
- 직장 내 상하 관계 수평적
- 보호자 및 환자가 간호사를 존중함 (컴플레인 거의 없음)
- 의료 사고 발생 시 병원과 노조가 간호사를 보호해 줌

개인적 결론:

↳ 한국은 번아웃이 빠르고 정신적 스트레스가 극심하지만, 뉴질랜드는 훨씬 안정적.

5 이민과 영주권 기회

뉴질랜드:

- 뉴질랜드는 간호사를 '필수 인력'으로 간주해서, 영주권 신청이 유리함.
- 간호사로 취업하면 곧바로 Work to Residence 비자를 받을 수 있음 (단기 영주권) → 2년 후 영구 영주권 가능.
- 영주권을 받으면 교육비, 의료 혜택, 연금 등 뉴질랜드 국민과 동일한 혜택을 받음.

솔직한 결론:

- 한국 간호사는 박봉 + 과로 + 태움 + 환자·보호자 갑질에 시달림
- 뉴질랜드 간호사는 적절한 업무량 + 높은 연봉 + 좋은 복지 + 삶의 질 보장
- 이민이 가능해 평안한 미래가 보장됨 (사람마다 평안한 미래의 기준은 다를수 있으니 고려바람)

뉴질랜드 이직을 고민하고 있다면 무조건 도전해볼 가치가 있다는걸 강조하고 싶어요. 물론 영어 준비와 면허 인증 과정이 필요하지만, 투자한 시간과 노력이 충분히 보상되는 환경이니 한번 진지하게 고려해보는 걸 추천합니다.

뉴질랜드 간호사의 연봉

뉴질랜드 간호사의 연봉은 다른 나라와 비교했을 때 다음과 같은 특징이 있습니다

🔖 호주와의 비교

초임 연봉:
- 뉴질랜드: NZ$79,000~(학사 졸업)
- 호주: NZ$88,000~(약 9,000 달러 더 높음)

최고 연봉:
- 뉴질랜드: NZ$111,000~
- 호주: NZ$120,000~(주에 따라 다름)

고위직 연봉:
- 뉴질랜드: 최대 NZ$133,000~
- 호주: 일부 주에서 NZ$200,000 이상 가능

🔖 한국과의 비교

환율을 고려했을 때(1 NZD = 800 KRW):
- 뉴질랜드 신규 간호사: 약 4,000만원 ~ 4,500만원
- 한국의 경우, 병원과 지역에 따라 다르지만 일반적으로 이보다 낮은 편입니다.

기타 특징

↝ 뉴질랜드는 2주마다 급여를 받는 주급제를 채택하고 있습니다.
↝ 기본 연봉 외에 야간, 주말, 공휴일 근무에 대한 추가 수당이 있습니다.
↝ 경력에 따라 연봉이 상승하는 구조를 가지고 있습니다.
↝ 미국 등 환율이 더 높은 국가에 비해서는 실질적인 수입이 낮을 수 있습니다.

결론적으로, 뉴질랜드의 간호사 연봉은 호주보다는 약간 낮지만, 한국보다는 높은 편입니다. 그러나 단순히 연봉만으로 비교하기보다는 생활비, 근무 환경, 사회적 지위 등을 종합적으로 고려해야 합니다.

Tapuhi Whai Rēhitatanga

Alternative titles for this job

Registered nurses assess, treat and support people who are sick, disabled or injured, in hospitals, clinics, rest homes, and nursing homes.

Pay

Enrolled nurses usually earn

$68K-$84K per year

Registered nurses usually earn

$74K-$153K per year

Source: Te Whatu Ora and NZNO, 2023 -2024

Job opportunities

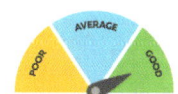

Chances of getting a job as a registered nurse are good due to high demand for their services

Length of training

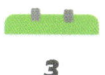

3

3 years of training required.

Pay

Pay for registered nurses varies depending on their qualification, experience, duties and responsibilities.

Enrolled nurses working for Te Whatu Ora Health NZ

- Graduate enrolled nurses working for Te Whatu Ora usually earn $68,000 a year. ($70,000 from 1 April 2024.)
- Enrolled nurses can earn $71,000 to $81,000. ($73,000 to $84,000 from 1 April 2024.)

Registered nurses working for Te Whatu Ora Health NZ

- Graduate registered nurses working for Te Whatu Ora usually earn $74,000 a year. ($76,000 from 1 April 2024.)
- Registered nurses usually earn $79,000 to $104,000. ($82,000 to $107,000 from 1 April 2024.)
- Senior registered nurses can earn $111,000 to $158,000. ($114,000 to $163,000 from 1 April 2024.)
- Nurse practitioners can earn $133,000 to $158,000 ($137,000 to $163,000 from 1 April 2024).

해외 간호사가
뉴질랜드 간호사가 되기 위한 조건

2024년 말부터 뉴질랜드 간호협회는 뉴질랜드 간호사가 되고자 하는 해외간호사들을 위해 새로운 제도를 도입하였습니다. 시간과 재정면에서 여러모로 이득이 될수 있는 제도라고 보여지고 합격 확률도 높은 것으로 현재 추정되고 있습니다.

그럼, 한국 간호사로서 뉴질랜드 간호사가 되기 위해 필요한 절차와 준비사항을 하나씩 살펴보겠습니다.

뉴질랜드 간호협회 요구사항

| Bachelor of Nursing 간호학사학위 | 1800시간 임상경력 | 공인인증 영어점수 |

기본 자격 요건 확인

뉴질랜드에서 간호사로 일하기 위해서는 뉴질랜드 간호사 등록위원회(NCNZ, Nursing Council of New Zealand)의 등록을

받아야 합니다. 이를 위해서는 다음과 같은 기본 자격 요건을 충족해야 합니다:

- 한국에서 인정된 간호학 학사 학위
- 한국 간호사 면허
- 최근 10년 1800시간 이상의 임상 경력
- 영어 능력(IELTS Academic 또는 OET 시험 성적 요구)

영어 능력 검증

뉴질랜드에서 간호사로 일하기 위해서는 영어 능력이 매우 중요합니다. NCNZ는 International English Language Testing System(IELTS: Academic module)또는 Occupational English Test(OET) 시험을 통해 영어 능력을 검증합니다. 일반적으로 요구되는 성적은 다음과 같습니다:

- **IELTS Academic:** 각 영역(듣기, 읽기, 쓰기, 말하기)에서 최소 7.0점 이상(쓰기 6.5 이상)

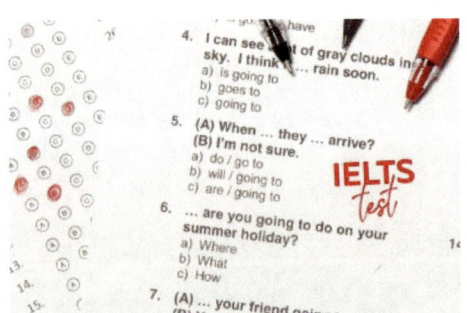

Listening	약 30분	문항 4개(Section)	40문제
Reading	약 60분	문항 4개(Section)	40문제
Writing	약 30분	문항 2개 Task	2 문제
Speaking	약 11분 ~ 14분	문항 3개 Part	

Or

↳ **OET:** 각 영역에서 최소 350등급 이상(쓰기 300점 이상)

과목	시험 시간	시험 내용
Listening	약 40분	총 42개 문항 Part A / 환자와 전문의의 상담 Part B / 직무 환경에서의 의료 관련 담화 Part C / 의학 강의, 강연
Reading	60분	총 42문제 빈칸 채우기, 학술지 및 논문에서 발췌된 긴 지문
Writing	45분	선택한 의료 분야에서 요구되는 소견서 및 진료 의뢰서 작성
Speaking	약 20분	선택한 의료 분야에서 일어날 수 있는 상황에 대한 Role Play

서류 준비 및 신청

NCNZ에 등록을 신청하기 위해서는 다음과 같은 서류를 준비해서 CGFNS(국제 간호사 자격 인증 기관)으로 보내야 합니다.

- ↳ **학위 증명서 및 성적 증명서**
- ↳ **학교 교육과정 실라부스**
- ↳ **한국 간호사 면허 증명서**
- ↳ **경력증명서**
- ↳ **영어 능력 시험 성적표**
- ↳ **범죄 기록 증명서(Police Clearance Certificate)**

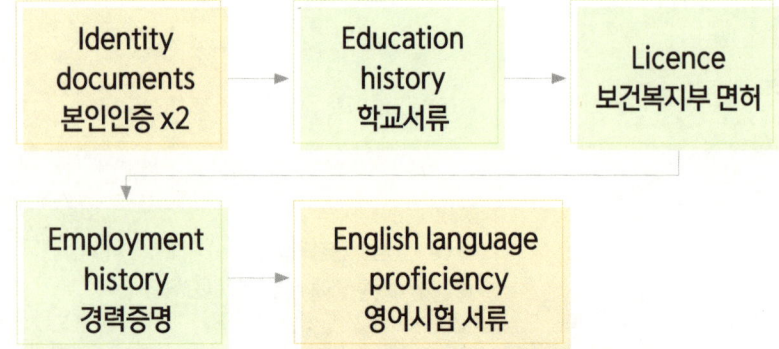

서류를 준비한 후, NCNZ의 온라인 포털을 통해 CGFNS에 먼저 등록 신청을 진행합니다.

CGFNS에서 서류 심사를 거치고 나면 결과 여부가 NCNZ로 넘어가며, NCNZ에서 또다시 자체의 서류 심사 과정이 진행됩니다. 이 과정은 신청자의 학교서류나 경력증명에 따라 몇주에서 몇 달이 소요될 수 있습니다.

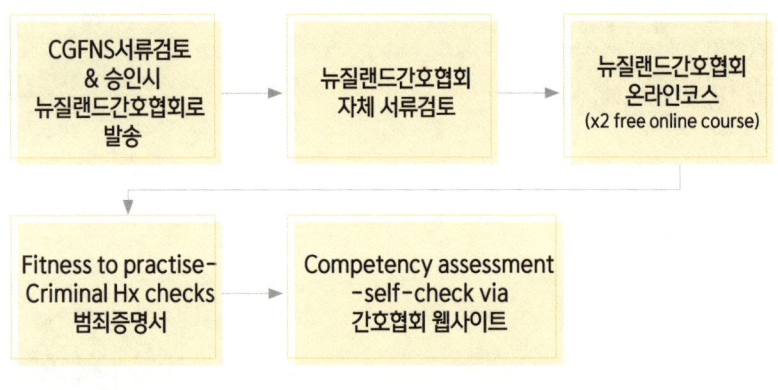

비용

- CGFNS: USD $ 300
- NCNZ: NZD $ 485
- International criminal history check: AUD $ 159
- Competence assessment examination(Theory NZD $ 140 + OSCE NZD $ 3500) cost vary but around NZD $ 4000

뉴질랜드 간호협회의 주요 변경 사항

⚘ Competence Assessment Programme(CAP) 대체:

보통은 NCNZ의 서류가 다 통과 되면 CAP코스를 하는 것이 통상적이었습니다. CAP는 뉴질랜드의 보건 시스템과 간호 실무에 익숙해지도록 돕는 프로그램으로, 일반적으로 몇 주에서 몇 달 정도 소요됩니다. CAP를 성공적으로 이수하면, 정식으로 간호사로 등록될 수 있었습니다. 하지만 이제 기존의 CAP코스는 더이상 필요하지 않고, 신청자는 온라인 이론 시험과 임상 실습 시험인 OSCE를 통과해야 합니다.

뉴질랜드 간호협회 웹사이트에는 이렇게 기재되어 있습니다.
: 2개의 뉴질랜드 온라인 코스를 수료해야 하고(무료 코스) , 실무적합성 검사(범죄 경력 증명서)를 제시해야 합니다. 그리고 competence assessment(이론시험과 OSCE 시험) 를 수행해야 하는지 필요하지 않은지 자가평가를 해야 합니다. 자가평가를 하게되면 한국 간호사는 무조건 이론시험과 OSCE를 수행해야 한다고 나옵니다.

Apply to the Nursing Council **AFTER** your documents are verified & complete the following:

↳ Welcome to Aotearoa New Zealand online courses

All nurses must complete two free online courses introducing you to culturally safe nursing practice in New Zealand.

↳ Fitness to practise checks

All nurses are required to undergo a criminal history check.

↳ Competence assessment

Some nurses will be required to undergo a competence assessment.

- Find out if you might require a competence assessment here.
- If you need a competence assessment, find out what that means here

You cannot apply directly to the Council as CGFNS must first verify your documents.

1. 이론 시험:

이론 시험은 온라인으로 진행되며, 전 세계의 Pearson VUE 시험 센터에서 응시할 수 있습니다.

한국현지 Pearson VUE는 아래 주소 입니다.

- **Pearson Professional Centers-Seoul, South Korea**
  Korea, South
  Seoul
  6F The Exchange Seoul,
  21 Mugyo-ro, Jung-gu,
  04520

이 시험은 **약물 시험과 간호 지식**을 평가하는 두가지 내용으로 구성됩니다.

- This is an online multi-choice examination that tests nursing knowledge, and it is taken at an accredited examination centre overseas or in New Zealand.
- Candidates complete 120 questions within 180 minutes.
- This examination is in two parts:
  - Part A: Medication Safety and
  - Part B: Nursing Knowledge
- You can have **three attempts** to successfully complete Parts A and B of the examination.
- On your first attempt, you must complete both Parts A and B.
- If you fail one part of the exam, you are only required to re-sit that part.
- The examination can only be taken at **Pearson VUE test centres** which are available in many countries.

이론 시험은 180 분 내에 120 문제를 풀어내야 합니다. 두가지 파트로 나뉘어 있는데 파트 A는 12개의 약물 안전성에 대한 문제이고 파트 B는 108개의 간호지식에 대한 문제입니다.

파트 A와 B 시험을 성공적으로 완료하기 위해 세 번의 시도가 허용됩니다. 첫 번째 시도에서는 반드시 파트 A와 B를 모두 완료해야 합니다. 시험의 한 파트를 실패한 경우, 해당 파트만 재응시하면 됩니다.

Your results will be available on your Pearson VUE dashboard soon after completion of an exam attempt.

The Nursing Council will communicate with you, within six weeks, when you have either passed both modules or you have used all your allocated three attempts. This communication will confirm your final result and outline next steps available to you.

시험 시도가 완료된 직후, 결과는 Pearson VUE 대시보드에서 확인할 수 있습니다.

뉴질랜드 간호협회는 두 모듈을 모두 통과했거나 할당된 세 번의 시도를 모두 사용한 경우, 6주 이내에 candidates에게 연락을 취합니다. 3번의 이론 시험에서 통과하지 못한 경우는 다시 뉴질랜드 간호협회에 등록을 하여 총 비용을 지급하고 처음부터 시험을 시도해야 합니다.

비용은 아래와 같습니다.(NZD)

Entire IQN exam fee	$ 140
Re-sit entire IQN exam fee	$ 140
Re-sit only Part A: Medication Safety Module	$ 32
Re-sit only Part B: Nursing Knowledge Module	$ 108

이론 시험 A파트와 B파트의 예시를 보자면 이러합니다.

• Part A : Medication Safety

Q1. A patient has been prescribed morphine 8mg 2-3hrly PRN for pain. Unit stock of morphine is 10mg/1ml. How much morphine should be drawn up for the patient?

Q2. A child weights 22.4kg, and the prescription is for 24mg/kg of body weight. The medication comes at a strength of 50mg/ml. how many mL of the medication should the child receive?

Q3. Ondansetron 2mg has been prescribed for a child who weights 13.6kg. The safe dosage of this drug is 0.15mg/kg. is 2mg a safe dose?

Q4. A patient is prescribed 250mg of antibiotics in 200mL of intravenous fluid over 30 minutes. The correct rate in mL per hour to set the infusion device is ?

• Part B : Nursing Knowledge

Q1. The role of the Nursing Council of New Zealand is

A : to protect the unregulated and regulated health workforce

B : to regulate doctors to protect public safety

C : to regulate nursing to protect public safety

D " to protect the nursing workforce

Q2. Prior to surgery, a patient is to have nothing to eat or drink. This is necessary to

A : assist in the proper absorption of the anaesthetic

B : prevent nausea and vomiting immediately after surgery

C : avoid the danger if inhaling the stomach contents

D : avoid incontinence during surgery

2. 임상 시나리오시험(OSCE):

OSCE는 뉴질랜드 내의 지정된 센터(크라이스트 처치 simulation assessment centre)에서 진행되며, 간호사의 임상 및 전문 기술을 테스트합니다. 시험 전에 이틀간의 Orientation Preparation course(OPC) 오리엔테이션 및 준비 과정이 제공됩니다.

이론 시험을 통과하고 OSCE를 치는 시기까지는 18개월의 기간이 주어집니다. OPC는 보통 OSCE 시험 일주일 전 정도에 진행됩니다.

- This is a **two-day orientation** and preparation course followed on a separate day by a **three-hour clinical examination** known as an Objective Structured Clinical Examination(OSCE).
- The orientation and preparation course and the OSCE take place in person at a Nursing Council-approved simulation & assessment centre in Christchurch, New Zealand.
- The OSCE assesses the candidate's applied nursing knowledge, communication, and safe clinical practice at the level of a New Zealand-registered nurse.

OSCE 시험에서는 120분 안에 10개의 시나리오(스테이션)를 완료해야 합니다. 각 스테이션당 12분이 배정되며, 이 중 2분은 지침 읽기에, 8분은 각 시나리오를 완료하는 데, 나머지 2분은 스테이션 간 이동에 사용됩니다 (스테이션당 2+8+2분).

OSCE에서 불합격할 경우, 최대 두 번 더 시험을 재응시할 수 있습니다.

오리엔테이션 및 준비 과정(OPC)과 OSCE는 크라이스트처치에 있는 Nurse Maude Simulation & Assessment Centre에서 진행됩니다.
https://www.nmsac.org.nz

- You must complete 10 OSCE scenarios(stations) in 120 minutes. Twelve minutes are allocated per station with two minutes for reading the instructions, eight minutes to complete each scenario and two minutes for movement between stations(2+8+2 minutes per station).
- If you do not pass the OSCE, you can re-sit the exam two more times.
- The orientation and preparation course and the OSCE are delivered by the Nurse Maude Simulation & Assessment Centre in Christchurch.?

한국 간호사로서 뉴질랜드 간호사가 되는 과정은 다소 복잡하고 시간이 걸릴 수 있지만, 철저한 준비와 노력을 통해 충분히 도전해볼 만한 가치가 있습니다. 뉴질랜드의 아름다운 환경과 양질의 의료 시스템 속에서 간호사로서의 커리어를 쌓고자 하는 분들에게 이 정보가 도움이 되었기를 바랍니다. 여러분의 도전을 응원합니다!

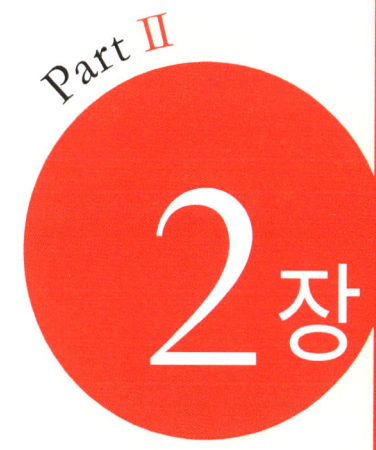

Part II

2장

10단계 예문과
**단계별 4개
연습 시나리오**

❶ 정신 건강 사정

Station 1: Mental Health Assessment

* Time: 10 minutes
* Setting: Post-operative care ward
* Patient: Mr. John Smith, 35 years old
* Presenting Complaint: depression and anxiety post operatively

✎ Example Scenario Description

Mr. John Smith, a 35-year-old male, was admitted following minor surgery. During routine postoperative care, Mr. Smith shared that he is experiencing feelings of depression and anxiety. He appears withdrawn and expresses difficulty sleeping since the procedure. As his nurse, you are tasked with conducting a mental health assessment to determine the severity of his symptoms, provide immediate emotional support, and develop a plan of care tailored to his needs.

> 존 스미스 씨(35세 남성)는 경미한 수술 후 입원했습니다. 수술 후 일반적인 간호 중, 스미스 씨는 우울감과 불안을 느낀다고 이야기했습니다. 그는 내성적인 모습을 보이며 수술 이후 수면에 어려움을 겪고 있다고 표현했습니다. 간호사로서, 당신은 그의 증상의 심각성을 평가하고 즉각적인 정서적 지원을 제공하며, 그의 필요에 맞춘 간호 계획을 수립해야 합니다.

Candidate Instructions:

1. Introduce Yourself and Explain the Assessment Process

- Approach Mr. Smith calmly and professionally, ensuring he feels comfortable and safe.
- Explain that you will ask some questions to better understand his emotional well-being and how you can support him during his recovery.
- Ensure that the conversation takes place in a private and quiet space to encourage openness and confidentiality.

> 스미스 씨에게 차분하고 전문적으로 접근하여 그가 편안하고 안전하다고 느낄 수 있도록 합니다. 그의 감정적 웰빙을 더 잘 이해하고 회복 과정에서 그를 어떻게 지원할 수 있는지 알기 위해 몇 가지 질문을 하겠다고 설명합니다. 대화가 개방적이고 개인정보 비밀이 유지될 수 있도록 조용하고 개인적인 공간에서 이루어지도록 합니다.

What to Say:

- "Hello, Mr. Smith, I'm [Your Name], one of the nurses looking after you today. I understand you've been feeling a bit down and anxious since your surgery. I'd like to ask you some questions about your emotional health so we can support you better. Is this a good time to talk?"

↳ "I want to assure you that everything you share will remain confidential within the care team. My goal is to help you feel more comfortable and supported."

- "안녕하세요, 스미스 씨. 저는 오늘 당신을 돌보는 간호사 [당신의 이름]입니다. 수술 후에 기분이 좀 가라앉고 불안감을 느끼고 계시다고 들었어요. 환자분의 감정 상태에 대해 몇 가지 질문을 드리고, 더 잘 지원해드리기 위해 노력하고 싶습니다. 지금 대화 나누기에 괜찮으신가요?"
- "환자분이 공유해주시는 모든 내용은 의료팀 내에서 비밀로 유지된다는 점을 안심시켜 드리고 싶습니다. 제 목표는 환자분이 더 편안하고 잘 지원받는다고 느끼실 수 있도록 돕는 것입니다."

---

2. Conduct a Comprehensive Mental Health assessment

2.1 Mood and Emotional State:

↳ Ask about his current mood and explore any feelings of sadness, anxiety, or hopelessness.

↳ Assess for signs of anhedonia(loss of interest in activities he usually enjoys).

- 현재 기분에 대해 물어보고 슬픔, 불안, 절망감 등의 감정을 살핍니다.
- 그가 보통 즐기던 활동에 흥미를 잃는 무쾌감(anhedonia) 징후가 있는지 평가합니다.

What to Say:

↳ "How have you been feeling emotionally since the surgery?"

↳ "Do you feel like you've lost interest in things you usually enjoy?"

"수술 이후로 감정적으로 어떻게 느끼셨나요?", "평소에 즐기던 것들에 흥미를 잃었다고 느끼시나요?"

2.2 Thought Processes and Perception:
- Inquire about any negative thoughts, feelings of guilt, or worthlessness.
- Ask if he has experienced any intrusive thoughts or unusual perceptions

- 부정적인 생각, 죄책감, 무가치감을 느낀 적이 있는지 질문합니다.
- 침투적 사고나 비정상적인 인식을 경험했는지 물어봅니다.

What to Say:
- "Have you been having any negative or distressing thoughts?"
- "Do you ever feel overwhelmed by feelings of guilt or worry?"

- "부정적이거나 괴로운 생각을 해본 적이 있나요?"
- "죄책감이나 걱정으로 압도당한 적이 있나요?"

2.3 Behaviour and Daily Functioning:
- Discuss how his emotional state is affecting his appetite, sleep, and energy levels.
- Ask about his ability to perform everyday tasks or maintain relationships.

- 그의 감정 상태가 식욕, 수면, 에너지 수준에 어떤 영향을 미치는지 논의하세요.
- 일상적인 작업을 수행하거나 인간관계를 유지하는 능력에 대해 물어보세요.

What to Say:

➢ "Have you noticed any changes in your appetite or sleep since the surgery?"

➢ "Do you feel like your energy levels have been lower than usual?"

"수술 이후 식욕이나 수면에 변화가 있었나요?", "에너지 수준이 평소보다 낮아진 것처럼 느껴지시나요?"

3. Risk Factors and Safety Assessment:

➢ Evaluate if he has experienced any thoughts of self-harm or suicide.

➢ Ask if he has a support system, such as family or friends, and determine their involvement in his recovery.

- 그가 자해나 자살에 대한 생각을 한 적이 있는지 평가합니다.
- 가족이나 친구와 같은 지지 체계가 있는지 물어보고, 그들이 그의 회복에 얼마나 관여하고 있는지 확인합니다.

What to Say:

➢ "Sometimes when people feel down, they may have thoughts of hurting themselves. Have you experienced any thoughts like that?"

➢ "Do you have friends or family members you can rely on for support?"

"가끔 사람들이 우울할 때 자신을 해치고 싶은 생각을 할 수도 있습니다. 그런 생각을 해본 적이 있으신가요?", "기댈 수 있는 친구나 가족이 있으신가요?"

4. Provide Emotional Support and Immediate Interventions

↠ Reassure him that his feelings are valid and that support is available.
↠ Offer relaxation techniques, such as deep breathing exercises, to help manage his anxiety.
↠ Suggest resources for further support, such as the hospital's mental health team or counselling services.

> 그의 감정이 정상적이며 지원이 가능하다는 점을 안심시켜 주세요.
> 심호흡 운동과 같은 이완 기법을 제공하여 불안을 관리하도록 도와주세요.
> 병원의 정신 건강팀이나 상담 서비스와 같은 추가 지원을 위한 자원을 제안하세요.

What to Say:

↠ "Thank you for sharing how you've been feeling. I want you to know that what you're going through is completely valid, and we're here to support you."
↠ "Would you like me to arrange a visit with our mental health specialist or a counsellor to talk further about what you're experiencing?"

> - "환자분의 감정을 함께 공유해 주셔서 감사합니다. 환자분이 겪고 있는 일이 완전히 정상적인 일임을 알려드리고 싶으며, 저희는 당신을 지원하기 위해 여기 있습니다."
> - "정신건강 전문가나 상담사와 만나서 현재 겪고 있는 일에 대해 더 이야기해보는 자리를 마련해 드릴까요?"

5. Notify the Healthcare Team and Develop a Plan of Care

- Document the findings of your assessment, including his reported symptoms, mood, and any identified risk factors.
- Notify the physician and mental health team for further evaluation if needed.
- Develop a plan of care that includes emotional support, monitoring, and referrals to appropriate services.

> 평가 결과를 문서화하여 환자가 보고한 증상, 기분, 그리고 확인된 위험 요인을 포함하십시오. 필요한 경우 추가 평가를 위해 의사와 정신건강 팀에 알리십시오. 정서적 지원, 모니터링, 그리고 적절한 서비스로의 의뢰를 포함하는 간호 계획을 수립하십시오.

What to Document:

"Mr. Smith reports feeling depressed and anxious since surgery, with difficulty sleeping and low energy levels. He denies thoughts of self-harm but expresses feelings of hopelessness. Will refer to the mental health team for further evaluation and provide ongoing emotional support."

Key Points to Remember:

- Ensure Mr. Smith feels heard and supported during the assessment.
- Assess mood, behavior, thought processes, and safety in a structured manner.
- Provide reassurance and practical resources for managing his emotional health.
- Collaborate with the healthcare team to ensure Mr. Smith receives comprehensive care.

Example Interaction:

Nurse: "Good morning, Mr. Smith. My name is [Nurse's Name], and I am one of the nurses here. I understand you've been feeling a bit down and anxious lately. Is it okay if we talk about how you've been feeling? This will help us understand what support you might need."

Mr. Smith: "Yes, that's fine. I've just been feeling really low and anxious since my surgery."

Nurse: "I'm sorry to hear that. Can you tell me more about your mood? How have you been feeling most of the time?"

Mr. Smith: "I've been feeling very down, like there's no point in anything. It's been going on for a few weeks now."

Nurse: "I understand. Have you noticed any changes in your sleep patterns or appetite recently?"

Mr. Smith: "Yes, I've had trouble sleeping, and I haven't been eating much."

Nurse: "Have you experienced any feelings of hopelessness or thoughts of harming yourself?"

Mr. Smith: "Sometimes I feel like I don't want to be here anymore, but I haven't made any plans."

Nurse: "Thank you for sharing that with me. It's really important that we address these feelings. I'm here to help, and we'll make sure you get the support you need."

Nurse: "Do you have any support from family or friends at the moment?"

Mr. Smith: "I do, but I haven't really talked to them about how I'm feeling."

Nurse: "It's good to know you have support available. We'll work together to help you feel better. I'll make a note of our conversation and suggest some steps we can take from here, including speaking with our mental health team."

✍ Documentation example

Date and Time

Patient states, "I feel down most of the time lately." Reports difficulty concentrating and a lack of interest in activities they used to enjoy. Denies hallucinations, delusions, or suicidal ideation. The patient describes issues with sleep and reduced appetite.

Patient appears well-groomed and is cooperative during the assessment. Eye contact was maintained throughout. Speech is clear and coherent with a normal rate and tone. Affect appears restricted but appropriate to the situation. No signs of agitation or psychomotor slowing were observed.

Patient presents with mild depressive symptoms, as evidenced by low mood, reduced interest, and difficulty concentrating. No immediate safety concerns were identified during the assessment.

Plan:
1. Provide reassurance and discuss available support options.
2. Refer to GP for evaluation and possible intervention for sleep and appetite concerns.
3. Follow-up in 2 weeks to monitor progress.
4. Encourage patient to use self-care strategies, such as relaxation techniques and engaging in physical activity.

Signature: Your name and designation

연습 Scenario 1:
Sadness and hopelessness

* Time: 10 minutes
* Setting: Emergency Department
* Patient: Mr. Mark Brown, 42 years old
* Presenting Complaint: Feelings of sadness and hopelessness

Example Scenario Description:

Mr. Mark Brown, a 42-year-old male, presents to the emergency department with complaints of persistent sadness, hopelessness, and a lack of motivation. He reports feeling overwhelmed by life stressors, including work-related pressures and personal challenges. He states that these feelings have worsened over the past few weeks, and he is having difficulty managing his emotions. Mr. Brown expresses concern about his mental health and is seeking support. As a nurse, you are tasked with conducting a mental health assessment to evaluate the severity of his symptoms and develop an appropriate plan of care.

✍ Candidate Instructions:

1. Introduce Yourself and Explain the Purpose of the Assessment

- ↳ Greet the patient and introduce yourself to establish rapport and trust.
- ↳ Clearly explain the purpose of the mental health assessment, assuring Mr. Brown that the goal is to understand his symptoms and provide appropriate care.

What to say:

- ↳ "Hello Mr. Brown, my name is [Your Name], and I'll be conducting a brief assessment today to better understand how you've been feeling. This will help us find the best way to support you and provide the care you need."
- ↳ "I know this may be difficult, but please know that everything we discuss is confidential, and I'm here to listen and help."

2. Conduct a Thorough Mental Health Assessment

- ↳ Ask open-ended questions to explore Mr. Brown's depressive symptoms, such as feelings of sadness, hopelessness, loss of interest, and changes in sleep or appetite.

- Inquire about any thoughts of self-harm or suicide, which is critical to assess in all cases of depression.
- Explore how these feelings have affected his daily functioning, work, and relationships.
- Assess for any physical symptoms related to depression, such as fatigue, changes in weight, or difficulty concentrating.

What to say:
- "Can you tell me more about how you've been feeling lately? Have there been specific moments when your sadness or hopelessness feels particularly overwhelming?"
- "Have you noticed any changes in your sleep, appetite, or energy levels during this time?"
- "I want to make sure you're safe, so can you tell me if you've had any thoughts of hurting yourself or if you've been thinking about not being here anymore?"
- "How are these feelings affecting your ability to get through daily tasks or interact with others?"

3. Document Findings and Develop a Plan of Care
- Document Mr. Brown's reported symptoms in detail, including the severity and duration of his feelings of sadness, hopelessness, and other associated symptoms.
- Note any risk factors for self-harm or suicide, and consider whether immediate intervention(e.g., referral

to mental health crisis services or suicide prevention protocols) is necessary.
- Develop an initial care plan that includes immediate emotional support, recommendations for therapy or counselling, and a follow-up plan for further evaluation.

What to say(for documentation):
- "I'll document your symptoms and concerns so we can keep track of what we've discussed and ensure you're receiving the right care. We'll also make a plan for follow-up support, including counselling and any other resources you may need."

4. Provide Immediate Support and Resources
- Reassure Mr. Brown that help is available, and that seeking support is an important step.
- Offer immediate coping strategies, such as relaxation exercises or grounding techniques, to help manage overwhelming feelings in the moment.
- Provide information on mental health services, including therapy options, and discuss potential medication management if appropriate.

What to say:
- "I understand this is really tough, but I want you to know that help is available, and we can work together to get you the support you need."
- "For now, let's take a moment to focus on your

breathing and practice a quick relaxation exercise. This can help ground you when things feel overwhelming."
- "We also have mental health professionals who can meet with you to explore further treatment options, whether that's therapy or medications. I can help arrange that for you."

5. Complete Documentation and Follow-Up Plan
- Ensure that Mr. Brown's mental health assessment is thoroughly documented, including any findings of depression, suicidal ideation, and the care plan developed.
- Provide a follow-up plan for further evaluation and ongoing support. Ensure Mr. Brown knows how to contact emergency services or mental health crisis support if his situation worsens.

What to say(for documentation):
- "I'll make sure to document everything we've discussed, including your symptoms, the immediate steps we've taken, and the follow-up plan. This will help ensure you receive the best care moving forward."

연습 Scenario 2:
Mood swings and erratic behaviour

* Time: 10 minutes
* Setting: Inpatient Psychiatric Unit
* Patient: Ms. Sarah Lee, 30 years old
* Presenting Complaint: Mood swings and erratic behaviour

✎ Example Scenario Description:

Ms. Sarah Lee, a 30-year-old female, has been admitted to the inpatient psychiatric unit due to severe mood swings and erratic behaviour. Over the past few weeks, her mood has fluctuated between extreme irritability and periods of intense euphoria, and she has demonstrated unpredictable behaviours such as impulsive actions and difficulty maintaining relationships. She has been finding it hard to control her emotions, and this has led to disruptions in her daily functioning. Your task is to conduct a thorough mental health assessment to evaluate the extent of her mood fluctuations and erratic behaviour and to develop an appropriate plan of care.

Candidate Instructions:

1. Introduce Yourself and Explain the Purpose of the Assessment

- Greet Ms. Sarah Lee in a calm, empathetic manner, ensuring a safe and supportive environment for her to express her concerns.
- Clearly explain the purpose of the mental health assessment and reassure her that you are there to help understand her symptoms and provide appropriate care.

What to say:
- "Hello Ms. Lee, my name is [Your Name], and I will be conducting a mental health assessment today to understand more about how you've been feeling. This will help us identify the best way to support you during your stay here."
- "I know it can be difficult to talk about your feelings, but I want you to know that everything you share with me is confidential, and I am here to listen and help."

2. Conduct a Thorough Mental Health Assessment Focusing on Mood and Behaviour

- Ask Ms. Lee open-ended questions to explore her

mood fluctuations, the intensity and duration of her symptoms, and any triggers or patterns she may have observed.
- Inquire about specific instances of erratic behaviour, such as impulsive decisions, aggression, or social withdrawal, and how these behaviours have impacted her life.
- Assess for any co-occurring symptoms, such as sleep disturbances, anxiety, or feelings of guilt, that could be contributing to her emotional state.
- Determine if Ms. Lee has any thoughts of self-harm or suicidal ideation, which is essential in any mental health assessment.

What to say:
- "Can you tell me more about how your mood has been shifting lately? Are there times when you feel more irritable or euphoric?"
- "Have there been any behaviours that you've noticed, like acting impulsively or making decisions you later regret?"
- "How have these mood swings and behaviours affected your relationships or your ability to manage daily activities?"
- "It's important to ask, have you had any thoughts about hurting yourself or anyone else during these times?"

3. Document Findings and Develop a Plan of Care

- Accurately document Ms. Lee's reported symptoms, including the severity, duration, and any possible triggers of her mood swings and erratic behaviors.
- Consider possible diagnoses based on her symptoms(e.g., Bipolar Disorder, Borderline Personality Disorder) and collaborate with the psychiatric team to confirm the diagnosis.
- Develop a plan of care that includes immediate emotional support, medication management(if applicable), and psychoeducation regarding managing mood swings.
- Ensure the plan addresses any safety concerns, including suicide prevention, and includes referrals to therapists or psychiatrists as needed.

What to say(for documentation):

- "I will document the details of your mood and behaviour, including what you've shared about any triggers, and work with our team to adjust your care plan accordingly."
- "We will ensure to support you in the best way possible and provide you with tools to manage your symptoms."

4. Provide Immediate Support and Resources

- Offer coping strategies to help Ms. Lee manage intense emotions, such as mindfulness exercises, breathing techniques, or grounding techniques to help her stay calm.
- Reassure Ms. Lee that her treatment plan will be tailored to her specific needs, which may include therapy, medication, or both.
- Provide information on the importance of ongoing therapy to help her better manage mood swings and improve her overall emotional well-being.

What to say:

- "I know this can be a challenging time for you, but we will provide you with the support you need. One way to manage these intense emotions is to practice deep breathing or mindfulness techniques, which can help calm your mind."
- "We will also ensure that you have access to the mental health professionals who can provide ongoing support, whether that's through therapy or medication."

5. Complete Documentation and Follow-Up Plan

- Ensure that all findings from the assessment are documented accurately, including Ms. Lee's mood patterns, behavior changes, and any co-occurring symptoms.

- ↠ Develop a follow-up plan that includes further psychiatric evaluation, medication review, and ongoing therapy sessions to help manage her symptoms.
- ↠ Ensure that safety measures are in place, including monitoring for any signs of self-harm or harm to others.

What to say(for documentation):

- ↠ "I'll make sure all the information we've discussed is documented, and we'll put together a plan to support your care moving forward. I'll also be checking in with you regularly to ensure you feel safe and supported."

연습 Scenario 3:
hearing voices and paranoid thoughts

* Time: 10 minutes
* Setting: Community Mental Health Clinic
* Patient: Mr. Alex Johnson, 25 years old
* Presenting Complaint: Hearing voices and paranoid thoughts

Example Scenario Description:

Mr. Alex Johnson, a 25-year-old male, has come to the community mental health clinic reporting auditory hallucinations(hearing voices) and paranoid thoughts. He describes hearing voices telling him that people are talking about him behind his back and believes that others are conspiring against him. He is feeling anxious and distressed about these symptoms and is finding it difficult to function in daily life. Your task is to conduct a thorough mental health assessment to evaluate the extent of his psychotic symptoms and develop an appropriate plan of care.

Candidate Instructions:

1. Introduce Yourself and Explain the Purpose of the Assessment

↪ Greet Mr. Johnson with a calm and empathetic approach to establish trust.
↪ Clearly explain the purpose of the mental health assessment and reassure him that you are there to understand his symptoms and provide support.

What to say:

↪ "Hello Mr. Johnson, my name is [Your Name], and I'm a nurse here. I'd like to talk to you about what you've been experiencing so we can understand your symptoms better and provide the right support for you."
↪ "I know these thoughts and voices can be unsettling, but I want you to know that we're here to help you through this."

2. Conduct a Thorough Mental Health Assessment Focusing on Psychotic Symptoms

↪ Ask Mr. Johnson about the nature of the voices he hears(e.g., are they familiar voices, do they give him commands, or just talk among themselves?).
↪ Inquire about the frequency, intensity, and content of the paranoid thoughts(e.g., what specific conspiracies or fears does he have?).

- Explore how these symptoms are affecting his daily life, social interactions, work, and sleep patterns.
- Assess for any other symptoms that could suggest a psychotic disorder, such as disorganized thinking, delusions, or withdrawal from reality.
- Screen for any co-occurring mood symptoms(e.g., depression, anxiety) or risk factors for self-harm or harm to others.

What to say:
- "Can you tell me more about the voices you're hearing? Are they saying anything specific to you?"
- "You mentioned feeling that people are conspiring against you. Can you explain what kind of situations make you feel this way?"
- "How have these experiences been affecting your daily activities or relationships with others?"
- "Do you ever feel like harming yourself or others because of these thoughts?"

3. Document Findings and Develop a Plan of Care
- Document Mr. Johnson's reported symptoms, including the content and frequency of the auditory hallucinations and paranoid thoughts.
- Include any relevant medical or psychiatric history, such as previous episodes of psychosis, substance use, or family history of mental health disorders.

- Develop a plan of care that includes crisis intervention(if necessary), referral to a psychiatrist for a full evaluation, and appropriate therapeutic support(e.g., cognitive-behavioural therapy for psychosis).
- Ensure the plan addresses any immediate safety concerns and outlines the next steps for treatment, such as medication options(e.g., antipsychotics) and follow-up appointments.

What to say(for documentation):
- "I'll document everything we've discussed, including the details of the voices you're hearing and your feelings of paranoia. This will help our team create the best treatment plan for you."
- "We will work together to address your symptoms and make sure you're safe during this time."

4. Provide Immediate Support and Resources
- Offer reassurance and validate Mr. Johnson's feelings, acknowledging how distressing psychotic symptoms can be.
- Introduce coping strategies, such as grounding techniques or reality testing, to help him manage distressing symptoms in the short term.
- Provide information on the role of medication in managing psychotic symptoms and discuss options for treatment.

↠ Ensure Mr. Johnson knows about available support services, such as peer support groups, case management, and ongoing therapy.

What to say:
↠ "It's important to know that you're not alone, and we will support you in managing these experiences. One way to help stay grounded is to focus on something in your environment, like a specific object, to help distract from the voices."
↠ "Medication can be very helpful for managing symptoms like this, and I'll make sure to discuss that with the doctor. We'll also provide you with ongoing support through therapy and community resources."

5. Complete Documentation and Follow-Up Plan
↠ Accurately document all findings from the assessment, ensuring to include the nature and severity of the psychotic symptoms and any associated factors.
↠ Outline a clear follow-up plan that includes psychiatric evaluation, medication management, and ongoing mental health support(e.g., therapy, case management).
↠ Ensure safety measures are in place, such as monitoring for any risks related to suicidal ideation or aggression.

What to say(for documentation):

➢ "I'll document all of your symptoms and ensure that we have a plan for you to meet with a psychiatrist soon. We'll also provide you with additional support and check in regularly."

연습 Scenario 4:
Flashbacks and nightmares

* Time: 10 minutes
* Setting: Veterans' Health Clinic
* Patient: Mr. Robert White, 40 years old
* Presenting Complaint: Flashbacks and nightmares related to combat experience

Example Scenario Description:

Mr. Robert White, a 40-year-old male, has come to the veterans' health clinic reporting frequent flashbacks and nightmares linked to his combat experience. He describes vivid, distressing memories of war, often accompanied by feelings of fear, helplessness, and anger. He has difficulty sleeping due to recurrent nightmares and experiences hypervigilance during the day. His symptoms have been impacting his daily functioning and relationships. Your task is to conduct a thorough mental health assessment to understand the extent of his symptoms and provide appropriate support, while also offering resources and treatment options for managing his post-traumatic stress disorder(PTSD).

Candidate Instructions:

1. Introduce Yourself and Explain the Purpose of the Assessment

- Greet Mr. White calmly and empathetically to establish rapport and trust.
- Clearly explain the purpose of the mental health assessment and reassure him that you are there to understand his symptoms and provide support.

What to say:

- "Hello Mr. White, my name is [Your Name], and I'm a nurse here. I'd like to talk with you today about what you've been experiencing, so we can understand how best to support you."
- "I know talking about your experiences can be difficult, but I want you to know that I'm here to listen and help you through this."

2. Conduct a Thorough Mental Health Assessment Focusing on PTSD Symptoms

- Ask Mr. White about the nature of his flashbacks and nightmares, including when they occur, how often, and how intense they are.

- Inquire about other symptoms of PTSD, such as hyperarousal(e.g., feeling easily startled, irritability), avoidance(e.g., avoiding places or people that remind him of combat), and negative mood(e.g., feelings of guilt or emotional numbness).
- Explore how these symptoms have impacted his ability to function in daily life, including work, relationships, and self-care.
- Ask about any coping mechanisms or strategies he has been using to manage his symptoms, including substance use or isolation.
- Assess for any thoughts of self-harm or suicidal ideation, as PTSD is associated with a higher risk for these behaviors.

What to say:
- "Can you tell me more about the flashbacks and nightmares you're experiencing? How often do they occur, and how do they make you feel?"
- "You mentioned feeling fearful and on edge during the day. Can you describe more about what that's like for you?"
- "Have you been avoiding any situations or places because of these memories?"
- "What kinds of things have you tried to cope with these feelings, and how have they been helping, if at all?"

↬ "Have you had any thoughts of harming yourself or feeling like things might be too much to handle?"

3. Document Findings and Develop a Plan of Care

↬ Document Mr. White's reported symptoms in detail, including the frequency, intensity, and duration of flashbacks, nightmares, and other PTSD-related symptoms.

↬ Include any relevant personal history, such as previous mental health diagnoses, traumatic events, and treatment history(e.g., prior counselling, medications).

↬ Develop a plan of care that includes a referral for a full psychiatric evaluation to formally diagnose and treat PTSD, considering options for trauma-focused therapies(e.g., Cognitive Behavioural Therapy for PTSD, Eye Movement Desensitization and Reprocessing) and medications(e.g., SSRIs or SNRIs).

↬ Address any immediate safety concerns, including providing resources for crisis management or a suicide prevention plan if applicable.

What to say(for documentation):
↬ "I'll document everything we've discussed today, including the frequency of your flashbacks and nightmares. This will help our team create a treatment plan tailored to your needs."

↠ "We'll make sure to connect you with additional resources, including therapy options and support groups for veterans, to assist you in managing these symptoms."

4. Provide Immediate Support and Resources

↠ Offer reassurance and validate Mr. White's experience, acknowledging the distressing nature of PTSD symptoms.
↠ Provide information about available therapeutic treatments, including individual therapy, group therapy, and medications that can help manage symptoms.
↠ Educate Mr. White on the importance of maintaining a support network, including connecting with other veterans or peer support groups.
↠ Discuss coping strategies that he can use in the interim to reduce distress, such as mindfulness exercises, deep breathing, and grounding techniques.

What to say:

↠ "I understand how overwhelming these experiences can be, and I want you to know that help is available. Therapy and medication can help you regain control and manage the flashbacks and feelings of distress."
↠ "We also have peer support groups for veterans where you can connect with others who understand what you're going through."

↳ "In the meantime, things like deep breathing and focusing on your surroundings can help ground you when these symptoms arise."

5. Complete Documentation and Follow-Up Plan
↳ Accurately document all findings, including Mr. White's symptoms, assessment of risk factors, and planned interventions.
↳ Ensure a clear follow-up plan, including scheduling an appointment with a psychiatrist or mental health specialist and providing information on crisis support services.
↳ Encourage Mr. White to reach out if he experiences an increase in symptoms or requires immediate assistance before the follow-up appointment.

What to say(for documentation):
↳ "We will follow up with you soon to assess how you're feeling and ensure that you have the necessary resources for managing your symptoms. Please don't hesitate to contact us if you need immediate help."

❷ 신체사정(활력징후 측정)

Station two: Physiological assessment

* Time: 10 minutes
* Setting: General practice clinic
* Patient: Mr. John Smith, 55 years old
* Presenting Complaint: Shortness of breath and persistent cough

✐ Example Scenario Description:

You are a registered nurse in a general practice clinic. Mr. John Smith, a 55-year-old male, has presented with complaints of shortness of breath and a persistent cough that has lasted for several weeks. He reports that his symptoms have gradually worsened, and he occasionally experiences chest tightness, especially at night. He has no known history of asthma but has been a smoker for 30 years. He denies any recent fever or upper respiratory infections but mentions that his sputum has been slightly discoloured.

Your task is to conduct a comprehensive respiratory assessment, identify any potential concerns, and determine the appropriate next steps for his care. You will need to evaluate his symptoms, perform a focused physical examination, and discuss a possible plan of care.

> 당신은 일반 진료 클리닉에서 근무하는 간호사입니다. 55세 남성인 John Smith 씨가 숨이 가쁘고 몇 주째 지속되는 기침 증상으로 내원했습니다. 그는 증상이 점차 악화되었으며, 특히 밤에 가슴이 조이는 느낌이 가끔 있다고 보고했습니다. 그는 천식 병력이 없지만, 30년 동안 흡연을 해왔습니다. 그는 최근에 열이나 상기도 감염 증상이 없었다고 부인하지만, 가래 색이 약간 변했다고 언급했습니다.
> Candidate의 임무는 포괄적인 호흡기 평가를 수행하여 잠재적인 문제를 파악하고 적절한 다음 단계를 결정하는 것입니다. 환자의 증상을 평가하고, 집중적인 신체 검사를 실시하며, 가능한 간호 계획을 논의해야 합니다.

Candidate Instructions:

1. Introduce Yourself and Establish Rapport

- Greet Mr. Smith warmly and introduce yourself.
- Explain the purpose of the assessment and ensure he is comfortable discussing his symptoms.
- Obtain consent before proceeding with the examination.

> Smith 씨에게 따뜻하게 인사하고 자신을 소개합니다. 평가의 목적을 설명하고, 증상에 대해 편안하게 이야기할 수 있도록 합니다. 검사를 진행하기 전에 동의를 받습니다

What to say:

"Hello, Mr. Smith, my name is [Your Name], and I am one of the nurses here today. I understand you have been experiencing shortness of breath and a persistent cough. I'd like to ask you some questions and conduct a respiratory assessment to better understand your condition. Does that sound okay to you?"

"Everything we discuss will remain confidential within the care team. My goal is to ensure we provide you with the best possible care."

> "안녕하세요, Smith 씨. 저는 오늘 여기에서 근무하는 간호사 [본인 이름]입니다. 숨이 가쁘고 지속적인 기침 증상이 있다고 들었습니다. 상태를 더 잘 이해하기 위해 몇 가지 질문을 드리고 호흡기 평가를 진행하고자 하는데 괜찮으신가요?"
> "우리가 나누는 모든 이야기는 의료 팀 내에서만 비밀로 유지됩니다. 저의 목표는 최상의 치료를 제공해 드리는 것입니다."

2. Conduct a Thorough Respiratory Assessment

2.1 History Taking

- Ask about the onset, duration, and progression of his symptoms.
- Determine any aggravating or relieving factors.
- Inquire about his smoking history and exposure to environmental irritants.
- Ask about past medical history, including any respiratory conditions or chronic diseases.
- Check for associated symptoms such as fever, wheezing, fatigue, or weight loss.

> - 증상의 시작 시기, 지속 기간 및 진행 상태에 대해 질문합니다.
> - 증상을 악화시키거나 완화하는 요인을 확인합니다.
> - 흡연력 및 환경적 자극물 노출 여부를 조사합니다.
> - 호흡기 질환이나 만성 질환 등 과거 병력을 확인합니다.
> - 발열, 천명(쌕쌕거림), 피로, 체중 감소 등의 관련 증상이 있는지 확인합니다.

What to say:

"Can you describe when your symptoms started and how they have changed over time?"

"Have you noticed anything that makes your breathing worse or better?"

"Do you have any history of respiratory conditions, such as asthma or chronic bronchitis?"

"Have you had any recent infections, fever, or night sweats?"

> "증상이 언제 시작되었고 시간이 지나면서 어떻게 변했는지 설명해 주시겠어요?"
> "호흡을 더 나빠지게 하거나 좋아지게 하는 요인이 있나요?"
> "천식이나 만성 기관지염 같은 호흡기 질환 병력이 있으신가요?"
> "최근에 감염이나 발열, 야간 발한을 경험한 적이 있으신가요?"

2.1 Physical Examination

- Measure and record vital signs, including respiratory rate, oxygen saturation, heart rate, and blood pressure.
- Observe for signs of respiratory distress, such as accessory muscle use, nasal flaring, or cyanosis.
- Perform auscultation of the lungs to assess for wheezing, crackles, or diminished breath sounds.
- Assess chest expansion and symmetry.
- Check for peripheral signs such as clubbing or cyanosis.

- 호흡수, 산소포화도, 심박수, 혈압 등 생명징후를 측정하고 기록합니다.
- 보조호흡 근육 사용, 코벌링임 증상, 청색증 등의 호흡곤란 징후를 관찰합니다.
- 폐의 청진을 통해 천명음, 기침소리, 또는 숨소리 감소 등을 사정합니다.
- 가슴 팽창 및 대칭을 평가합니다.
- 손톱끝 변형이나 청색증을 확인하여 말초혈관 상태를 봅니다.

What to say:

↪ "I'm going to check your vital signs and listen to your lungs to assess how well you're breathing."

↪ "Take a deep breath in and out for me, please. Let me know if you feel any discomfort."

"저는 이제 생명징후를 확인하고, 호흡이 잘 되고 있는지 평가하기 위해 폐소리를 들을 거예요.", "깊게 숨을 들이쉬고 내쉬어 주세요. 불편한 느낌이 있으면 말씀해 주세요."

3. Document Findings and Develop a Plan of Care

↪ Record all assessment findings, including reported symptoms, physical examination results, and any risk factors identified.

↪ Notify the physician if there are signs of respiratory compromise or potential underlying conditions such as COPD or pneumonia.

↪ Provide initial management recommendations, such as smoking cessation support, breathing exercises, or inhaler use if appropriate

↪ Arrange for further diagnostic tests, such as a chest X-ray, pulmonary function tests, or sputum analysis if indicated.

- 보고된 증상, 신체검사 결과, 식별된 위험 요소 등을 포함한 모든 평가 결과를 기록합니다.
- 호흡 기능 저하나 COPD, 폐렴과 같은 잠재적인 기저 질환의 징후가 있을 경우 의사에게 알립니다.
- 적절하다면 흡연 중단 지원, 호흡 운동, 흡입기 사용 등의 초기 관리 권장 사항을 제공합니다.
- 필요한 경우 흉부 엑스레이, 폐 기능 검사, 객담 분석과 같은 추가 진단 검사를 준비합니다.

What to say:

↳ "Based on my assessment, I will document my findings and discuss them with the physician. They may recommend further tests or treatments."

↳ "Since you mentioned a history of smoking and persistent symptoms, we may consider additional tests to check your lung function."

↳ "Would you like some information on smoking cessation programs and breathing exercises that might help improve your symptoms?"

"제가 진행한 사정을 바탕으로 찾아낸 사항을 문서화하고 의사와 논의할 예정입니다. 의사분들이 추가 검사나 치료를 권할 수 있습니다.", "흡연 경력과 지속적인 증상을 언급하셨기 때문에, 폐 기능을 확인하기 위한 추가 검사를 고려할 수 있습니다.", "흡연 중단 프로그램이나 증상 개선에 도움이 될 수 있는 호흡 운동에 대한 정보를 원하시면 알려드릴 수 있습니다."

Documentation example

Date/Time

Patient presented with complaints of shortness of breath(SOB) and a persistent cough lasting approximately two weeks. He reports the cough is dry and worse at night. Denies chest pain, fever, or recent illnesses. States SOB is more noticeable during physical activity, such as walking up stairs. No history of asthma or known lung conditions. Smokes approximately 10 cigarettes per day for the last 30 years.

Vital Signs; for example,
- Temperature: 36.8°C
- Pulse: 92 bpm, regular
- Respiratory Rate: 22 breaths/min
- Blood Pressure: 138/86 mmHg
- SpO2: 94% on room air

Physical Examination; for example,
- Inspection: Mild dyspnea noted; no cyanosis or accessory muscle use.
- Palpation: Equal chest expansion bilaterally; no tenderness.
- Percussion: Resonant sounds bilaterally.
- Auscultation: Bilateral lung fields clear; no wheezes, crackles, or rhonchi.

Assessment; for example,
- Persistent dry cough and mild dyspnoea on exertion.
- Oxygen saturation slightly decreased.
- Potential contributing factors: smoking history and possible environmental irritants.

Plan:
1. Educate patients on smoking cessation resources and the impact of smoking on respiratory health.
2. Recommend chest X-ray to rule out underlying conditions(e.g., chronic obstructive pulmonary disease, interstitial lung disease).
3. Provide a prescription for a short-term bronchodilator if symptoms persist.
4. Suggest saline nasal spray or humidifier for nighttime symptom relief.
5. Advise follow-up appointment in one week to reassess symptoms and discuss test results.
6. Encourage increased fluid intake and rest.

Signature: name, RN

연습 Scenario 1:
Abdominal pain and nausea

* Time: 10 minutes
* Setting: Inpatient Medical Unit
* Patient: Mr. David Lee, 45 years old
* Presenting Complaint: Abdominal pain and nausea

Example Scenario Description:

Mr. David Lee, a 45-year-old male, presented to the inpatient medical unit with complaints of abdominal pain and nausea that started earlier in the day. The pain is described as crampy and intermittent, located in the lower abdomen. He mentions feeling bloated and having difficulty eating due to nausea. Your task is to conduct a thorough gastrointestinal assessment to identify potential issues, such as gastrointestinal infection, obstructive conditions, or gastrointestinal disorders, and develop an appropriate care plan.

Candidate Instructions:

1. Introduce Yourself and Explain the Purpose of the Assessment

- Greet Mr. Lee and introduce yourself, explaining the reason for your assessment.
- Let the patient know that you will ask a series of questions and perform an examination to better understand the cause of his symptoms.

What to say:

- "Hello Mr. Lee, my name is [Your Name], and I'm a nurse here on the inpatient medical unit. I understand you're experiencing abdominal pain and nausea. I'm going to ask you a few questions and perform an exam to help determine what might be causing these symptoms, so we can provide the best care possible, is that ok with you"

2. Perform a Thorough Gastrointestinal Assessment

History Taking:

- Ask about the onset, duration, and nature of the abdominal pain(e.g., dull, crampy, sharp) ? Use COLDSPA pain assessment framework

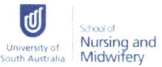

COLDSPAA
Symptom Analysis Mnemonic

Mnemonic	Question
Character	Describe the sign or symptom (feeling, appearance, sound, smell or taste if applicable)
Onset	When did it begin?
Location	Where is it? Does it radiate? Does it occur anywhere else?
Duration	How long does it last? Does it recur?
Severity	How bad is it? How much does it bother you?
Pattern	What makes it better or worse?
Associated factors / how it **A**ffects the pt	What other symptoms occur with it? How does it affect you?

Table 2-3 taken from:
Lewis, P and Foley, D 2011, *Weber & Kelly's Health Assessment in Nursing*, Lippincott Williams & Wilkins Pty Ltd, a division of Wolters Kluwer Health, NSW.

- Inquire about any changes in bowel habits(e.g., diarrhoea, constipation, blood in stools).
- Ask about any recent dietary changes, recent travel history, or potential exposure to infections.
- Assess for other symptoms, such as fever, vomiting, weight loss, or changes in appetite.
- Inquire about his medical history, including any previous gastrointestinal issues(e.g., ulcers, IBS, history of gallstones, surgeries).

Physical Examination:

- Inspect the abdomen for distention, scars, or visible abnormalities.
- Palpate the abdomen to assess for tenderness, rigidity, or masses.

- Percuss the abdomen for signs of fluid or gas accumulation.
- Auscultate bowel sounds to assess for normal, hypoactive, or hyperactive bowel sounds.
- Perform a digital rectal exam if indicated(e.g., for patients with possible constipation or rectal bleeding).

Key Questions to Ask:
- "Can you describe the pain? Is it sharp, crampy, or dull?"
- "Where exactly is the pain located? Does it radiate anywhere?"
- "Have you noticed any changes in your bowel habits, like diarrhoea or constipation?"
- "Have you had any recent changes in your diet or any new foods that could have caused this?"
- "Are you feeling nauseous all the time, or does it come and go? Have you vomited?"
- "Have you experienced any weight loss, fever, or blood in your stool?"

3. Document Findings and Develop a Plan of Care
- Document Mr. Lee's symptoms, including the onset, quality, and location of the abdominal pain, along with any associated symptoms such as nausea, bloating, and changes in bowel habits.

- Record the results of the physical examination, including tenderness, abnormal bowel sounds, or other findings.
- Include any relevant medical history and potential risk factors.
- Suggest possible next steps for diagnosis, including laboratory tests(e.g., CBC, liver function tests, stool cultures), imaging studies(e.g., abdominal ultrasound, CT scan), and consultations(e.g., gastroenterologist).
- Prepare for interventions such as IV fluids, antiemetics, or pain management, depending on the findings.

What to say(for documentation):
- "Patient reports intermittent crampy abdominal pain localized to the lower abdomen for the past 6 hours, associated with nausea. No vomiting or changes in bowel habits. Physical exam: mild tenderness to palpation in the lower abdomen, normal bowel sounds. No signs of fever or weight loss. Plan: CBC, abdominal ultrasound, IV fluids, and antiemetics as needed."

4. Communicate Findings and Plan of Care
- Share the findings with the physician and other relevant team members to ensure the appropriate tests and interventions are initiated.
- Update Mr. Lee on the next steps, explaining any tests or treatments that will be provided.

What to say to the patient:
- "Mr. Lee, I've completed your assessment, and we'll be doing some tests, including blood work and an ultrasound, to help us figure out what's causing your abdominal pain. I will keep you updated on the results and what we can do to help you feel better."

5. Complete Documentation and Follow-Up Plan
- Ensure that all findings, assessments, and interventions are documented clearly in the patient's record.
- Outline the follow-up plan, including scheduled tests, treatments, and when to follow up with the physician.
- Ensure all necessary orders are placed(e.g., labs, imaging, medication orders).

What to say(for documentation):
- "Follow-up with results of abdominal ultrasound and labs, including liver function tests. Anticipating pain management and possible IV fluids based on test outcomes. Gastroenterology consult if needed."

연습 Scenario 2:
Headaches and dizziness

* Time: 10 minutes
* Setting: Neurology Outpatient Clinic
* Patient: Ms. Linda Green, 50 years old
* Presenting Complaint: Headaches and dizziness

✏ Example Scenario Description:

Ms. Linda Green, a 50-year-old female, has presented with complaints of persistent headaches and dizziness that have been occurring for the past few weeks. She describes her headaches as moderate in intensity, throbbing in nature, and localized to the temples. The dizziness is associated with light-headedness and occasional balance issues. Your task is to perform a thorough neurological assessment to identify any potential neurological causes for her symptoms and provide appropriate care.

Candidate Instructions:

1. Introduce Yourself and Explain the Purpose of the Assessment

- Greet Ms. Green and introduce yourself, explaining that you will be performing a neurological assessment to better understand the cause of her symptoms.
- Ensure the patient is comfortable and informed throughout the process.

What to say:

- "Hello Ms. Green, my name is [Your Name], and I am a nurse here in the neurology outpatient clinic. I understand that you have been experiencing headaches and dizziness. I'm going to perform a neurological assessment to help determine what might be causing these symptoms and guide the next steps in your care."

2. Perform a Thorough Neurological Assessment

History Taking:

- Ask about the onset, frequency, duration, and characteristics of the headaches(e.g., throbbing, sharp, constant, intermittent)- Use COLDSPA framework
- Inquire about any associated symptoms, such as nausea, visual disturbances, or sensitivity to light or sound.

- Ask about the nature of the dizziness(e.g., light-headedness, vertigo, balance problems) and if it occurs with any specific activities or movements.
- Determine if there is any history of head trauma, neurological conditions, or family history of migraines or stroke.
- Review any recent changes in medication or lifestyle(e.g., stress, sleep patterns, diet).

Physical Examination:
- Assess the patient's vital signs, including blood pressure, heart rate, respiratory rate, and temperature.
- Perform a cranial nerve examination to assess the function of the 12 cranial nerves(e.g., checking for pupillary response, facial symmetry, and visual fields).
- Conduct a motor and sensory examination to check for strength, coordination, and sensation.
- Perform a cerebellar examination to assess coordination, balance, and gait.
- Perform a Romberg test to assess for balance issues related to dizziness.

Key Questions to Ask:
- "When did your headaches start, and how often do they occur?"

- "Can you describe your headache? is it throbbing, sharp, or dull?"
- "Do you have any other symptoms with the headaches, like nausea, vision changes, or light sensitivity?"
- "Can you explain what you mean by dizziness? Do you feel lightheaded, or is it more of a spinning sensation?"
- "Have you had any recent changes in your daily routine, stress levels, or sleep patterns?"
- "Do you have a history of headaches or any neurological conditions, like migraines or stroke, in your family?"

3. Document Findings and Develop a Plan of Care

- Record Ms. Green's symptoms, including the characteristics and frequency of her headaches, and any associated symptoms such as dizziness, visual changes, or nausea.
- Document the results of the physical and neurological examination, noting any abnormal findings such as changes in coordination, balance, or cranial nerve function.
- Develop an initial plan of care, including the need for further investigations such as imaging studies(e.g., MRI or CT scan), laboratory tests(e.g., blood tests to rule out infections or anemia), and possibly a referral to a neurologist for a comprehensive evaluation.

What to say(for documentation):

↳ "Patient reports moderate, throbbing headaches localized to the temples, occurring 3-4 times per week for the past 3 weeks, associated with occasional light-headedness and balance issues. No visual disturbances, nausea, or vomiting noted. Physical examination shows normal cranial nerve function and no signs of neurological deficits. Plan: MRI of the brain, blood tests for anemia and electrolyte imbalances, referral to neurology for further evaluation."

4. Communicate Findings and Plan of Care

↳ Share the findings with the physician and other relevant team members to ensure the appropriate tests and interventions are initiated.

↳ Update Ms. Green on the next steps, explaining any further tests or treatments that will be provided.

What to say to the patient:

↳ "Ms. Green, based on our assessment, we would like to do an MRI to rule out any neurological causes for your headaches and dizziness. I'll also arrange for some blood tests to check for anaemia or other possible causes. We'll be sure to follow up with you on the results, and in the meantime, we can discuss treatment options to manage your symptoms."

5. Complete Documentation and Follow-Up Plan

- Ensure that all findings, assessments, and interventions are documented clearly in the patient's record.
- Outline the follow-up plan, including scheduled tests, treatments, and when to follow up with the physician.
- Ensure all necessary orders are placed(e.g., imaging, lab tests, neurology referral).

What to say(for documentation):

- "Follow-up with results of MRI and blood tests. Plan for a referral to neurology for further evaluation. Discussed the potential treatment options for headache management, including over-the-counter medications and stress reduction techniques."

연습 Scenario 3:
Joint pain and swelling

* Time: 10 minutes
* Setting: Orthopaedic Outpatient Clinic
* Patient: Mr. Michael Davis, 35 years old
* Presenting Complaint: Joint pain and swelling

Example Scenario Description:

Mr. Michael Davis, a 35-year-old male, has come to the orthopaedic outpatient clinic with complaints of joint pain and swelling, particularly in his knees and wrists. He reports that the symptoms have been worsening over the past month and that the swelling is accompanied by stiffness, especially in the mornings. He has difficulty performing daily activities such as walking and typing at work. Your task is to perform a musculoskeletal assessment to understand the severity of his symptoms and develop an appropriate plan of care.

Candidate Instructions:

1. Introduce Yourself and Explain the Purpose of the Assessment

- Greet Mr. Davis, introduce yourself, and explain that you will be conducting a musculoskeletal assessment to understand the cause of his joint pain and swelling.
- Ensure the patient is comfortable and encourage open communication about his symptoms.

What to say:

- "Hello Mr. Davis, my name is [Your Name], and I'm a nurse here in the orthopaedic outpatient clinic. I understand that you've been experiencing joint pain and swelling. I'll be conducting a thorough assessment to help determine the cause of your symptoms and discuss the next steps in your care, is that ok with you"

2. Perform a Thorough Musculoskeletal Assessment

History Taking:

- Ask about the onset, duration, and severity of his joint pain and swelling.
- Inquire whether the pain is constant or intermittent and whether it is aggravated or relieved by any specific activities.
- Ask about any history of trauma or injury to the affected joints.

- Determine if he has any other symptoms such as fever, fatigue, or weight loss that may suggest an inflammatory or systemic condition.
- Review any family history of musculoskeletal diseases such as arthritis or autoimmune conditions.
- Ask about any previous treatments or medications used for the joint pain and their effectiveness.

Physical Examination:
- Inspect the affected joints for signs of swelling, redness, and deformities.
- Palpate the joints to assess for tenderness, warmth, and any abnormal masses.
- Assess the range of motion(ROM) for each joint, noting any limitations or pain during movement.
- Perform specific tests for joint stability, such as the McMurray test for the knee or the Phalen's test for the wrist, if applicable.
- Check for signs of systemic involvement, such as rashes or swollen lymph nodes.
- Perform a neurovascular assessment, including checking pulses and capillary refill in the affected limbs.

Key Questions to Ask:
- "When did your joint pain start, and how long has it been bothering you?"
- "Is the pain constant, or does it come and go? Is it

worse at any particular time of day?"
- "Are the joints swollen? Do you notice any redness or warmth around the joints?"
- "Do you have any other symptoms like fever, weight loss, or fatigue?"
- "Have you had any recent injuries or falls that could have contributed to the pain?"
- "Do you have a family history of arthritis, autoimmune conditions, or joint problems?"

3. Document Findings and Develop a Plan of Care

- Record Mr. Davis's symptoms, including the onset, severity, and location of the pain and swelling.
- Document the results of the physical examination, noting any abnormalities such as joint swelling, reduced range of motion, or tenderness.
- Develop an initial care plan, which may include recommendations for pain management, diagnostic testing(e.g., X-rays, blood tests for inflammation markers), and referrals to specialists(e.g., rheumatology or orthopaedics) if necessary.
- Suggest potential treatment options such as anti-inflammatory medications, physical therapy, or joint protection techniques.

What to say(for documentation):
- "Patient presents with joint pain and swelling, particularly in the knees and wrists, for the past

month. Swelling is associated with morning stiffness and worsens with activity. No history of trauma noted. Physical exam reveals mild swelling in bilateral knees and wrists, with reduced range of motion in both joints. Plan: Order X-rays of the affected joints, CBC, and ESR to evaluate for inflammation. Refer to orthopaedics for further management."

4. Communicate Findings and Plan of Care

↠ Share your findings with the physician and discuss the next steps, including any necessary tests or referrals.

↠ Update Mr. Davis on the next steps, explaining the diagnostic tests and treatments you plan to initiate.

What to say to the patient:

↠ "Mr. Davis, based on our assessment, we'll be ordering some X-rays of your knees and wrists to get a better idea of what might be causing the swelling and pain. We will also check some blood tests to assess for inflammation. Depending on the results, we may refer you to a specialist for further treatment, which could include physiotherapy or medications to manage the pain and inflammation."

5. Complete Documentation and Follow-Up Plan

↠ Ensure that all findings, assessments, and interventions are clearly documented in the patient's record.

- Outline the follow-up plan, including the necessary tests, referrals, and a timeline for follow-up care.
- Ensure that all orders are placed, and the patient is scheduled for the appropriate follow-up visits.

What to say(for documentation):
- "Follow-up with X-ray and lab results. If results indicate inflammatory or degenerative conditions, refer to orthopaedic or rheumatology specialist. Advise patient on joint protection techniques and pain management options, including over-the-counter anti-inflammatory medications."

연습 Scenario 4:
Sudden onset of right-sided weakness

* Time: 10 minutes
* Setting: Medical Ward
* Patient: Mr. James Wilson, 45 years old
* Presenting Complaint: Sudden onset of right-sided weakness

Example Scenario Description:

Mr. James Wilson, a 45-year-old male, has presented to the medical ward with a sudden onset of right-sided weakness and difficulty speaking. He is alert but appears distressed and reports that the symptoms began approximately 30 minutes ago. You are tasked with performing a comprehensive neurological assessment to identify any neurological deficits and escalate care if necessary.

✍ Candidate Instructions:

1. Introduce Yourself and Explain the Purpose of the Assessment

↪ Greet Mr. Wilson, introduce yourself, and explain the purpose of the neurological assessment.
↪ Ensure the patient feels comfortable and understands the process.

What to say:

↪ "Hello Mr. Wilson, my name is [Your Name], and I'm a nurse here on the medical ward. I understand that you're experiencing weakness on your right side and difficulty speaking. I'm going to perform a neurological assessment to help us understand what's happening and make sure you get the appropriate care, is that ok with you."

2. Perform a Comprehensive Neurological Assessment

Level of Consciousness(LOC):

↪ Assess Mr. Wilson's level of consciousness using the AVPU scale(Alert, Verbal, Pain, Unresponsive) or Glasgow Coma Scale(GCS).
↪ Note any changes in his alertness or responsiveness.

What to check for:

↪ Is the patient alert and oriented to person, place, time, and situation?
↪ Any signs of confusion or drowsiness?

What to say:
➢ "Can you tell me your name, where you are right now and what date it is?"

Cranial Nerve Assessment:

- Check for facial symmetry(e.g., ask the patient to smile or puff out both cheeks).
- Assess speech clarity by asking the patient to repeat simple phrases(e.g., "The sky is blue").
- Listen for slurring or difficulty pronouncing words.

What to check for:
- Any facial drooping or asymmetry?
- Is speech clear, or does it sound slurred?

What to say:
- "Can you smile for me?"
- "Can you say, 'The sky is blue'?"

Limb Strength Testing:

- Assess the strength of both upper and lower limbs, comparing the right side to the left side.
- Ask the patient to push or pull against your hands and check for any weakness or inability to perform movements.

What to check for:
- Any noticeable weakness or inability to perform tasks with the right side?

What to say:
- "Please push your hands against mine as hard as possible."
- "Now, push your feet against my hands."

Sensory Assessment:

- Perform a sensory assessment by lightly touching the skin on both sides of the patient's body and asking if there are differences in sensation.
- Ask the patient to close their eyes and describe the sensation as you touch different areas on both sides of the body.

What to check for:
- Any differences in sensation between the right and left sides of the body?

What to say:
- "Can you tell me if you feel the same on both sides of your body?"

3. Measure and Document Vital Signs

→ Measure the patient's vital signs, including blood pressure, heart rate, oxygen saturation, and respiratory rate.

→ Document the vital signs and note any abnormal findings, particularly if the blood pressure is elevated or oxygen saturation is low.

What to check for:

→ Are there any abnormalities in the vital signs that could indicate a potential stroke or other neurological issue?

4. Document Findings and Escalate Care if Necessary

→ Document all findings from the neurological assessment, including LOC, cranial nerve function, limb strength, and sensory assessments.

→ If any significant abnormalities are found(e.g., signs of a stroke or neurological deficit), escalate care immediately. Notify the physician and prepare for further imaging or intervention as required.

What to document:

→ "Patient presents with sudden right-sided weakness and difficulty speaking. Neurological exam shows decreased strength on the right side with mild facial asymmetry. Speech is slightly slurred. Vital signs: BP 190/110, HR 98, O2 saturation 94%. Immediate escalation for stroke workup ordered. CT scan to be performed."

5. Communicate with the Team

- Notify the physician about the patient's condition, discussing your findings and the need for further diagnostic tests, such as a CT scan or MRI.
- Ensure that the medical team is aware of the potential urgency of the situation.

What to say to the physician:
- "Mr. Wilson is presenting with sudden right-sided weakness, slurred speech, and elevated blood pressure. I have performed a neurological exam and noted decreased strength and facial asymmetry. I recommend immediate imaging to rule out a stroke. Please advise on the next steps."

6. Follow-Up and Plan

- Ensure the patient is closely monitored and that further diagnostic tests are completed as soon as possible.
- Provide the patient with emotional support, explaining that the medical team is working quickly to determine the cause of his symptoms.

What to say to the patient:
- "Mr. Wilson, we are taking your symptoms very seriously, and we're going to perform some tests to better understand what's going on. We'll keep you updated, and you'll be closely monitored."

❸ 세부 생리학적 사정

Specific physiological assessment

* Time: 10 minutes
* Setting: Orthopaedic Surgical Ward
* Situation: Recognizing and assessing symptoms of Deep Vein Thrombosis(DVT) and Pulmonary Embolism (PE)

✐ Example Scenario Description:

You are a registered nurse working in an Orthopaedic Surgical ward. Your patient, Mrs. Sarah Thompson, a 65-year-old female, has recently undergone total knee replacement surgery and has been immobile for a few days. She is now experiencing pain and swelling in one of her legs, along with shortness of breath. You suspect she may be experiencing symptoms of DVT and/or PE, and you must assess the patient appropriately.

Your task is to effectively assess the patient's symptoms, perform the necessary physiological assessments to detect DVT or PE, and communicate with the medical team about the findings.

당신은 정형외과 외과 병동에서 근무하는 간호사입니다. 당신의 환자인 사라 톰슨(Sarah Thompson) 씨는 65세 여성으로, 최근 무릎 전치환술(total knee replacement) 수술을 받았으며, 며칠 동안 움직이지 못했습니다. 현재 그녀는 한쪽 다리에 통증과 부종을 호소하며, 숨이 가쁜 증상을 보이고 있습니다. 당신은 그녀가 심부정맥혈전증(DVT) 및/또는 폐색전증(PE)의 증상을 보이고 있다고 의심하며, 환자의 상태를 적절하게 평가해야 합니다.

간호사로써 당신의 임무는 환자의 증상을 효과적으로 평가하고, DVT 또는 PE를 감지하기 위한 필요한 생리학적 평가를 수행하며, 의료진에게 소견을 전달하는 것입니다.

Candidate Instructions:

Step 1: Patient Communication and Preparation

1.1 Introduce Yourself and Confirm Identity

- Knock on the door, greet the patient, and check their identity.

What to say:

- "Good morning, Mrs. Thompson. My name is [Your Name], and I am your nurse today. Could you please confirm your full name and date of birth? Thank you."

좋은 아침입니다, 톰슨 씨. 저는 오늘 담당 간호사 [본인의 이름]입니다. 성함과 생년월일을 확인해 주시겠어요? 감사합니다."

1.2 Explain the Procedure and Obtain Consent

- Explain the importance of assessing for symptoms of DVT and PE, as well as the physical examination you will perform.

What to say:

- "I need to check your legs for signs of a condition called deep vein thrombosis, which can cause swelling, pain, and redness. I'll also assess your breathing and listen to your chest to rule out pulmonary embolism. You may feel a bit of pressure during the exam, but it shouldn't be painful. Do you have any questions or concerns before we begin?"

> "다리에서 부종, 통증, 발적을 유발할 수 있는 심부정맥혈전증(DVT) 징후가 있는지 확인해야 합니다. 또한 폐색전증(PE)을 배제하기 위해 호흡 상태를 평가하고 가슴 소리를 청진할 것입니다. 검사 중 약간의 압력을 느낄 수 있지만 통증이 있지는 않을 것입니다. 시작하기 전에 궁금한 점이나 걱정되는 사항이 있으신가요?"

: Obtain verbal consent before proceeding.

1.3 Ensure Patient Comfort and Positioning

↣ Ask the patient to lie down or sit comfortably, ensuring their legs are accessible for examination.

What to say:

↣ "Please lie back in bed so I can examine your legs and listen to your chest."

Step 2: Equipment Preparation and Aseptic Technique

2.1 Perform Hand Hygiene and Wear PPE

↣ Wash hands thoroughly and wear gloves if necessary. Ensure aseptic technique if touching any areas of potential infection or injury.

> 손을 깨끗이 씻고 필요하면 장갑을 착용합니다. 감염이나 부상의 위험이 있는 부위를 만질 경우 무균 기술을 유지해야 합니다.

What to say:
- ⤳ "I'm now washing my hands and putting on gloves to ensure cleanliness during the exam."

Step 3: Assessment of Deep Vein Thrombosis (DVT)

3.1 Inspect the Leg for Signs of DVT
- ⤳ Inspect the affected leg for signs of redness, swelling, or any visible distended veins. DVT usually occurs in the lower extremities.

> **심부정맥혈전증(DVT) 징후에 대한 다리 검사**
> 영향을 받은 다리를 검사하여 발적, 부기 또는 확장된 정맥이 보이는지 확인합니다. DVT는 일반적으로 하체에서 발생합니다.

What to say:
- ⤳ "I'm going to inspect your legs to check for any signs of redness, swelling, or visible veins."

> "다리에 발적, 부기 또는 확장된 정맥이 있는지 확인하기 위해 검사를 진행하겠습니다."

3.2 Palpate the Leg for Tenderness
- ⤳ Gently palpate along the calf, thigh, and ankle for any areas of tenderness, warmth, or swelling. Be sure to use your fingers to avoid unnecessary pressure.

> 종아리, 허벅지, 발목을 따라 부드럽게 촉진하여 압통, 따뜻한 감각 또는 부기가 있는지 확인합니다. 불필요한 압력을 피하기 위해 손가락을 사용하여 검사합니다.

What to say:

↠ "I will gently palpate your leg to see if you feel any tenderness or warmth, which can be a sign of clotting."

"다리에 부드럽게 촉진하여 압통이나 따뜻한 감각이 있는지 확인하겠습니다. 이는 혈전의 징후일 수 있습니다."

3.3 Perform the Homan's Sign Test

↠ Flex the patient's foot upward towards the shin while the leg is extended. This maneuver may provoke pain if DVT is present, although this test is not always reliable.

호만 징후 검사를 수행합니다.
환자의 다리를 편 상태에서 발을 정강이 쪽으로 위로 굽힙니다. 이 동작이 통증을 유발하면 DVT가 있을 가능성이 있지만, 이 검사는 항상 신뢰할 수 있는 것은 아닙니다.

What to say:

↠ "I'm going to gently flex your foot upward to check for any pain, which could be a sign of deep vein thrombosis."

"제가 발을 부드럽게 위로 굽혀서 통증이 있는지 확인하겠습니다. 통증이 느껴진다면 심부정맥혈전증의 징후일 수 있습니다."

Step 4: Assessment for Pulmonary Embolism (PE)

4.1 Assess for Shortness of Breath (SOB)
- Ask the patient if they are experiencing any shortness of breath, especially when resting or during mild exertion.

환자에게 휴식 중이거나 가벼운 활동 중에 숨이 차는 느낌이 있는지 물어보세요.

What to say:
- "Are you feeling short of breath, especially when you're lying down or after minimal activity?"

"누워 있을 때나 가벼운 활동 후에 숨이 차는 느낌이 드시나요?"

4.2 Inspect the Chest for Tachypnoea
- Observe the patient's breathing rate for signs of tachypnoea (rapid breathing), which may indicate difficulty breathing due to PE.

환자의 호흡 속도를 관찰하여 빈호흡(빠른 호흡) 징후가 있는지 확인합니다. 이는 폐색전증(PE)으로 인한 호흡 곤란을 나타낼 수 있습니다.

What to say:
- "I'm checking your breathing rate to see if it's faster than normal, which can sometimes happen with pulmonary embolism."

"폐색전증이 있을 때 호흡이 평소보다 빨라질 수 있기 때문에 지금 호흡 속도를 확인하겠습니다."

4.3 Measure Oxygen Saturation

↘ Use a pulse oximeter to measure oxygen saturation. A low oxygen saturation level may indicate PE.

펄스 옥시미터를 사용하여 산소 포화도를 측정하겠습니다. 낮은 산소 포화도는 폐색전증을 나타낼 수 있습니다.

What to say:

↘ "I'm going to check your oxygen levels now to ensure you're breathing adequately."

"이제 산소 수치를 확인하여 충분히 호흡하고 계신지 확인하겠습니다."

4.4 Auscultate the Lungs

↘ Listen to the patient's lungs for abnormal breath sounds, such as crackles or wheezing, which may indicate a PE. A clear lung sound does not rule out PE, but it is important to rule out other potential causes.

환자의 폐에서 이상 호흡음(수포음 또는 천명음 등)이 있는지 확인합니다. 폐색전증이 있더라도 폐음이 정상일 수 있지만, 다른 가능한 원인을 배제하는 것이 중요합니다.

What to say:

↘ "I'm going to listen to your lungs to make sure there are no abnormal sounds that might suggest a pulmonary issue."

"폐에 이상 소리가 있는지 확인하기 위해 청진하겠습니다."

Step 5: Post-Assessment Care and Patient Education

5.1 Dispose of Used Equipment Properly
- Dispose of any gloves, tissues, or swabs used during the assessment into the appropriate waste container.

사용한 장갑, 휴지 또는 면봉을 적절한 폐기물 용기에 버리십시오.

What to say:
- "I'm disposing of any used materials now to maintain cleanliness."

"지금 사용한 물품들을 처분하여 청결을 유지하겠습니다."

5.2 Monitor for Changes or Complications
- Encourage the patient to notify you if they experience sudden chest pain, worsening shortness of breath, or calf pain.

환자에게 갑작스러운 흉통, 악화되는 호흡곤란 또는 종아리 통증이 발생하면 즉시 알리도록 권장하세요.

What to say:
- "Please let me know immediately if you experience sudden chest pain, increased shortness of breath, or if the pain in your leg gets worse."

"갑작스러운 흉통, 호흡곤란이 심해지거나 다리 통증이 악화되면 즉시 알려주세요."

5.3 Provide Patient Education on Symptoms to Monitor

⇾ Educate the patient on the importance of monitoring for signs of complications, including chest pain, difficulty breathing, or swelling in the legs.

> 환자에게 흉통, 호흡곤란 또는 다리 부종과 같은 합병증의 징후를 지속적으로 관찰하는 것이 중요하다고 교육합니다.

What to say:

⇾ "Keep an eye on your symptoms. If you start to feel worse, especially with sudden shortness of breath, chest pain, or significant swelling in your legs, seek immediate medical attention."

> "증상을 주의 깊게 살펴봐 주세요. 갑작스러운 호흡곤란, 흉통 또는 다리의 심한 부종이 나타나면 즉시 의료진에게 연락하시거나 병원을 방문하세요."

Step 6: Documentation and Reporting

6.1 Document the Findings and Patient Response

⇾ Record the findings of your DVT and PE assessment, including any positive signs (e.g., swelling, redness, pain, shortness of breath, oxygen saturation, lung auscultation).

Example Documentation:

⇾ "Patient assessed for DVT and PE. Right leg showed signs of swelling, tenderness, and warmth, suggestive of possible DVT. O2 saturation measured at 94%, no abnormal breath sounds on auscultation. Patient reports mild shortness of breath. Monitoring and follow-up recommended."

6.2 Report Any Abnormal Findings

➢ If any red flags are identified (e.g., signs of PE, DVT), report these findings to the medical team immediately for further investigation.

What to say:

➢ "I've documented my findings and will report any concerning signs to the medical team for further evaluation."

연습 Scenario 1:
Ileus Symptoms Management for Post-Colectomy Patient

* Time: 10 minutes
* Setting: Surgical Ward
* Situation: Ileus Symptoms Management for Post-Colectomy Patient

Example Scenario Description:

You are a registered nurse working in a Surgical ward. Your patient, Mr. Daniel Hayes, is a 72-year-old male who underwent a colectomy for colon cancer. He is experiencing symptoms of ileus, including nausea & vomiting, abdominal bloating, distension, and a lack of bowel sounds. Your task is to assess the ileus symptoms and perform a thorough physiological evaluation to monitor for any complications, such as bowel obstruction or peritonitis.

Candidate Instructions:

Step 1: Patient Communication and Preparation

1.1 Introduce Yourself and Confirm Identity

➣ Knock on the door, greet the patient, and confirm their identity.

What to say:

➣ "Good morning, Mr. Hayes. My name is [Your Name], and I'm your nurse today. Could you please confirm your full name and date of birth for me? Thank you."

1.2 Explain the Situation and Obtain Consent

➣ Explain the nature of ileus, the symptoms, and the importance of monitoring and assessment.

What to say:

➣ "I understand you are experiencing some bloating and discomfort in your abdomen with nausea & vomiting. This could be due to ileus, a condition where the bowel temporarily stops moving after surgery. I will need to assess your abdomen and check for other signs to make sure we monitor your recovery. Is it okay if I perform a quick examination of your abdomen?"

: Obtain verbal consent before proceeding.

1.3 Ensure Patient Comfort and Positioning

➣ Ensure the patient is in a comfortable position, preferably supine, with their head slightly elevated, allowing access to the abdominal area for assessment.

What to say:

↝ "Please lie back comfortably while I check your abdomen. I'll adjust your position if needed."

Step 2: Equipment Preparation and Aseptic Technique

2.1 Perform Hand Hygiene and Wear PPE

↝ Wash hands thoroughly and wear gloves. If necessary, wear an apron and mask for additional precaution.

What to say:

↝ "I'm now washing my hands and wearing gloves to ensure we maintain cleanliness while I perform the assessment."

Step 3: Abdominal Assessment and Monitoring for Ileus Symptoms

3.1 Abdominal Inspection and Palpation

↝ Inspect the abdomen for visible signs of distension, bloating, or abnormal swelling. Gently palpate the abdomen to assess for tenderness, guarding, or rigidity, which could suggest other complications like peritonitis.

What to say:

↝ "I'm going to gently check your abdomen for any swelling or tenderness. Please let me know if you feel any pain."

3.2 Assess Bowel Sounds

➤ Using a stethoscope, listen to all four quadrants of the abdomen for bowel sounds. Ileus typically presents with absent or hypoactive bowel sounds.

What to say:

➤ "I'm listening to your bowel sounds now. With ileus, the bowel sounds may be absent or weak. Let me know if you feel any discomfort."

3.3 Assess for Tenderness or Guarding

➤ Press gently on the abdomen to check for signs of tenderness or rigidity, which could indicate peritonitis or another underlying issue requiring immediate attention.

What to say:

➤ "I'm pressing gently on your abdomen to check for any unusual tenderness. Let me know if it feels painful or uncomfortable."

Assessment techniques

Order of examination always IPPA:

Inspection
Palpation
Percussion
Auscultation

**EXCEPT Abdominal Assessment = Inspection, Auscultation, Palpation, Percussion

Step 4: Physiological Assessment and Monitoring

4.1 Monitor Vital Signs

⇢ Measure the patient's blood pressure, heart rate, respiratory rate, and temperature. Pay attention to signs of hypovolemia, such as low blood pressure and elevated heart rate, or any signs of systemic infection like a fever.

What to say:

⇢ "I'm checking your vital signs now. This helps us ensure that your body is responding well to recovery and that we're staying ahead of any complications."

4.2 Assess for Signs of Shock

⇢ Monitor for any signs of shock, such as a rapid heart rate, low blood pressure, or cool extremities, which may indicate poor perfusion or other issues like sepsis.

What to say:

⇢ "Please let me know if you feel dizzy, faint, or lightheaded. These could be signs of low blood pressure or other changes we need to monitor."

4.3 Observe for Peritonitis or Complications

⇢ Watch for any new signs of peritonitis, such as persistent or worsening abdominal pain, increased tenderness, or changes in abdominal rigidity, which may signal infection.

What to say:

↪ "I'm assessing for any signs of infection or peritonitis, which could cause increased pain or rigidity in your abdomen. If you feel more pain, please let me know immediately."

Step 5: Management and Post-Procedure Care

5.1 Provide Pain Relief

↪ If the patient reports discomfort or pain, provide appropriate analgesia or comfort measures as per the protocol.

What to say:

↪ "I understand this procedure may be uncomfortable. If you need anything for the pain, just let me know, and I can arrange for something to help."

5.2 Monitor for Worsening Symptoms

↪ Continue to monitor the patient's condition for any changes in symptoms, such as increased bloating, abdominal pain, or signs of bowel obstruction or peritonitis.

What to say:

↪ "We will keep monitoring your symptoms closely. If you notice any new or worsening pain, or if the bloating increases, please inform me immediately."

5.3 Educate the Patient on Ileus Management

↝ Explain how the patient can manage symptoms at home, including the importance of avoiding solid food until bowel function returns, and watching for signs of complications.

What to say:

↝ "Once you're discharged, it's important to avoid heavy meals until your bowel function returns. If you notice any increasing pain, fever, or no bowel movement after a few days, please contact us right away."

Step 6: Documentation and Reporting

6.1 Document the Procedure and Patient Response

↝ Record the time and date of the abdominal assessment, the condition of the abdomen (distension, tenderness, bowel sounds), and any changes noted in the patient's symptoms.

Example Documentation:

↝ "Abdominal assessment completed for patient Mr. Daniel Hayes. Abdomen distended with hypoactive bowel sounds. Mild tenderness noted on palpation. Vital signs: BP 120/75, HR 85, Temp 37.3°C. No signs of peritonitis or shock. Patient reports moderate discomfort. Persistent nausea and vomiting bile, Monitoring ongoing."

6.2 Report Any Abnormal Findings

- If any abnormal findings are observed, such as signs of bowel obstruction or worsening symptoms, report them to the medical team immediately for further evaluation and management.

What to say:

- "I've documented the assessment and will report any significant changes to the medical team for further evaluation."

연습 Scenario 2:
Increased Intracranial Pressure (ICP) Symptoms Post-Craniotomy Surgery

* Time: 10 minutes
* Setting: Neuro - Surgical Ward
* Situation: Assessment of Increased Intracranial Pressure (ICP)

Example Scenario Description:

You are a registered nurse working in a neuro-surgical ward. Your patient, Mrs. Emily Thompson, a 45-year-old female, has recently undergone a craniotomy for the removal of a brain tumor. Post-operatively, the patient shows signs of increased intracranial pressure (ICP), including headache, altered consciousness, and potential changes in pupil size. Your task is to assess the symptoms of increased ICP and perform a thorough physiological evaluation to monitor for any complications, such as brain herniation or worsening neurological status.

Candidate Instructions:

Step 1: Patient Communication and Preparation

1.1 Introduce Yourself and Confirm Identity
↳ Knock on the door, greet the patient, and confirm their identity.

What to say:
↳ "Good morning, Mrs. Thompson. My name is [Your Name], and I'm your nurse today. Could you please confirm your full name and date of birth? Thank you."

1.2 Explain the Situation and Obtain Consent
↳ Explain the importance of monitoring for signs of increased ICP and the need for a neurological assessment.

What to say:
↳ "I understand you've had surgery recently to remove a brain tumor. I need to assess you for signs of increased intracranial pressure (ICP), which could happen after surgery. This will involve checking your alertness, eyes, and some other signs. Are you comfortable with that?"

: Obtain verbal consent before proceeding.

1.3 Ensure Patient Comfort and Positioning
↳ Ensure the patient is lying in a semi-recumbent position (30-45 degrees) to reduce ICP and make the assessment easier.

What to say:

↪ "Please lie back in a comfortable position, I'll help you with your pillow if you need. I'm going to check a few things to make sure everything is okay."

Step 2: Equipment Preparation and Aseptic Technique

2.1 Perform Hand Hygiene and Wear PPE

↪ Wash hands thoroughly and wear gloves.

What to say:

↪ "I'm now washing my hands and putting on gloves to ensure everything stays clean while I perform the assessment."

Step 3: Assessment of Symptoms and Neurological Examination for ICP Increase

3.1 Assess the Patient's Level of Consciousness

↪ Use the Glasgow Coma Scale (GCS) to assess the patient's level of consciousness. Look for any signs of deterioration or confusion. A GCS score less than 8 may indicate severe impairment.

What to say:

↪ "I'll be checking how alert you are by asking a few questions and checking your responses. Just respond when you feel comfortable."

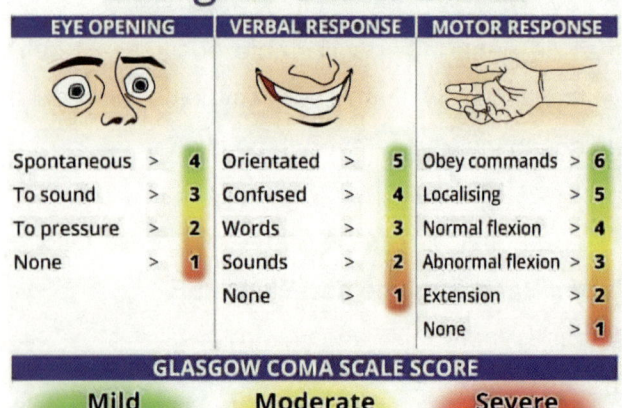

3.2 Assess Pupil Response

↠ Check the size and reaction of the pupils to light using a penlight. Unequal, fixed, or dilated pupils may indicate increased ICP or impending brain herniation.

What to say:

↠ "I'm going to shine a light in your eyes to check your pupils' reaction. It may feel a little bright, but it won't take long."

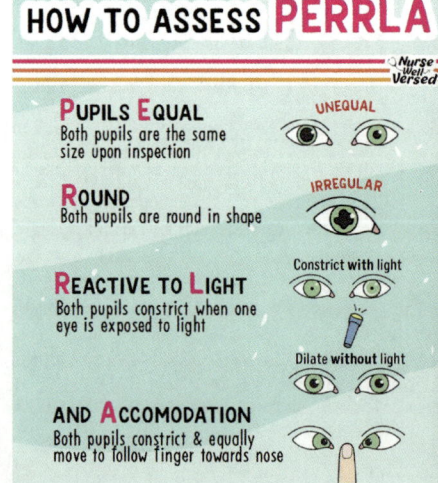

3.3 Check for Signs of Headache or Nausea

↣ Ask the patient if they are experiencing a headache or nausea, which are common symptoms of increased ICP. A worsening headache or nausea/vomiting can suggest that ICP is rising.

What to say:

↣ "Are you feeling any pain or pressure in your head right now, or do you feel nauseous at all?"

3.4 Assess for Other Signs of ICP Increase

↣ Check for signs such as confusion, agitation, or changes in speech or motor function. Monitor for signs of brainstem compression, such as irregular breathing patterns.

What to say:

↣ "I'll also be checking for any signs of confusion or changes in your speech. Let me know if you feel any difference in how you're thinking or speaking."

Step 4: Physiological Monitoring and Specific ICP Assessments

4.1 Monitor Vital Signs

↣ Measure the patient's blood pressure, heart rate, respiratory rate, and temperature. Increased ICP may cause high blood pressure with a widening pulse pressure (systolic increases, diastolic remains the same or decreases) and bradycardia (slowed heart rate). A decreased respiratory rate may also be observed.

What to say:
- "I'm going to check your vital signs now to make sure everything is within normal limits."

4.2 Assess for Cushing's Triad
- Look for signs of Cushing's Triad (a late sign of ICP increase), which includes hypertension (increased systolic blood pressure), bradycardia (slow heart rate), and irregular respirations (Cheyne-Stokes or apnea).

What to say:
- "I'm closely monitoring your vital signs, as changes in your blood pressure, heart rate, or breathing can tell us a lot about how your brain is responding."

4.3 Assess Respiratory Pattern
- Observe the patient's respiratory pattern. Irregular or abnormal breathing patterns (e.g., Cheyne-Stokes or Biot's respiration) may indicate increased pressure on the brainstem.

What to say:
- "I'll be watching your breathing pattern closely to see if there are any changes. If you notice anything unusual in your breathing, let me know immediately."

Step 5: Management and Post-Procedure Care

5.1 Provide Pain Relief and Comfort

- If the patient reports a headache or discomfort, administer prescribed pain relief as per protocol. Ensure the head of the bed remains elevated to reduce ICP.

What to say:

- "Let me know if you feel any pain, and I'll make sure you get something for that. I'm also keeping your head elevated to help with the pressure."

5.2 Positioning for ICP Management

- Ensure the head of the bed is elevated at 30-45 degrees, as this can help decrease ICP by promoting venous drainage from the brain.

What to say:

- "I'm adjusting your bed slightly to make sure your head is elevated. This position helps reduce the pressure on your brain."

5.3 Monitor for Worsening Symptoms

- Continue to monitor the patient for any signs of deterioration, including changes in consciousness, breathing pattern, or pupil response. Notify the medical team immediately if worsening symptoms are observed.

What to say:

⤳ "We'll keep a close watch on your symptoms. If anything changes or gets worse, please let me know immediately."

Step 6: Documentation and Reporting

6.1 Document the Assessment and Findings

⤳ Record the time and date of the neurological assessment, the GCS score, pupil size and reaction, vital signs, and any reported symptoms (e.g., headache, nausea). Document any changes in the patient's condition.

Example Documentation:

⤳ "Neurological assessment completed for patient Mrs. Emily Thompson. GCS score 15, pupils equal and reactive to light. No headache or nausea reported. Vital signs: BP 130/85, HR 72, RR 16, Temp 37.2°C. No signs of ICP increase or herniation observed at this time."

6.2 Report Abnormal Findings to Medical Team

⤳ If there are any signs of increased ICP, report them to the attending physician or the surgical team for immediate intervention.

What to say:

⤳ "I've documented the findings and will report any significant changes in your condition to the medical team right away."

✱ Study Tips!!

- Practice performing neurological assessments, including the Glasgow Coma Scale and pupil response.
- Familiarize yourself with the early and late signs of increased ICP.
- Focus on the patient's comfort and clarity in explaining assessments to reduce anxiety.
- Time yourself during practice to ensure a thorough, efficient assessment.
- Review protocols for managing increased ICP and recognize signs requiring immediate intervention.

연습 Scenario 3:
Hyponatremia (Na 113) Post-Total Knee Replacement

* Time: 10 minutes
* Setting: Orthopaedic Surgical Ward
* Situation: Assessment of Hyponatremia Symptoms Post-Total Knee Replacement

✏ Example Scenario Description:

You are a registered nurse working in the Orthopaedic Surgical ward. Your patient, Mr. Robert Harris, a 67-year-old male, has recently undergone a total knee replacement (TKR) surgery. Post-operatively, his sodium level has dropped to 113 mmol/L, a condition known as hyponatremia. You are tasked with assessing his symptoms and performing a thorough physiological assessment to monitor for complications such as neurological changes, confusion, or seizures due to the low sodium level.

Candidate Instructions:

Step 1: Patient Communication and Preparation

1.1 Introduce Yourself and Confirm Identity

↠ Knock on the door, greet the patient, and confirm their identity.

What to say:

↠ "Good morning, Mr. Harris. My name is [Your Name], and I'm your nurse today. Could you please confirm your full name and date of birth? Thank you."

1.2 Explain the Situation and Obtain Consent

↠ Explain the importance of monitoring for symptoms of hyponatremia and the need for a thorough assessment.

What to say:

↠ "I see that your sodium levels are low, which can sometimes cause symptoms like confusion, headache, or weakness. I'll be checking your mental status, vital signs, and looking for any signs that might suggest you're feeling unwell because of the low sodium. Are you comfortable with that?"

: Obtain verbal consent before proceeding.

1.3 Ensure Patient Comfort and Positioning

↠ Ensure the patient is in a comfortable position, preferably lying flat or slightly elevated in bed, to facilitate your assessment.

What to say:
- "Please make yourself comfortable, Mr. Harris. I'll just take a few minutes to check your symptoms and ensure everything is okay."

Step 2: Equipment Preparation and Aseptic Technique

2.1 Perform Hand Hygiene and Wear PPE
- Wash hands thoroughly and wear gloves if required.

What to say:
- "I'm washing my hands and putting on gloves to ensure the procedure is sterile and clean."

Step 3: Assessment of Symptoms and Physiological Examination for Hyponatremia

3.1 Assess the Patient's Level of Consciousness
- Check the patient's level of consciousness, using the Glasgow Coma Scale (GCS) to detect any signs of confusion, drowsiness, or decreased responsiveness, which may indicate worsening hyponatremia.

What to say:
- "Mr. Harris, I'll be asking you a few questions to make sure everything is clear in your mind. Just answer when you feel comfortable."

3.2 Monitor for Neurological Symptoms
- Ask the patient if they are feeling any dizziness, confusion, nausea, or headache, as these are

common signs of hyponatremia. Severe hyponatremia can lead to seizures or even coma.

What to say:

↳ "Are you feeling dizzy, confused, or having any trouble concentrating? Any headaches or nausea?"

3.3 Check for Weakness or Fatigue

↳ Ask the patient if they are experiencing any muscle weakness or fatigue. Weakness, especially in the extremities, can indicate severe hyponatremia.

What to say:

↳ "Do you feel weak in your arms or legs, or have any trouble moving around?"

3.4 Perform a Full Neurological Examination

↳ Assess the patient's pupils (size and reaction to light), speech, and motor function. Look for any signs of cerebral Oedema, such as unequal pupils or abnormal reflexes.

What to say:

↳ "I'll be checking your pupils to see how they react to light and making sure your reflexes are normal. Please tell me if anything feels unusual."

Step 4: Physiological Monitoring and Specific Assessments for Hyponatremia

4.1 Measure Vital Signs

↳ Measure the patient's blood pressure, heart rate,

respiratory rate, and temperature. Low sodium levels can cause hypotension, tachycardia, and altered respiratory patterns.

What to say:
↳ "I'm going to take your vital signs now to see if there's anything unusual with your blood pressure or heart rate."

4.2 Monitor for Seizures or Cerebral Oedema
↳ Observe for signs of seizure activity (twitching, jerking movements) or any abnormal posturing. Hyponatremia can lead to cerebral oedema, which increases the risk for seizures. Notify the physician if any seizure-like activity is observed.

What to say:
↳ "Let me know if you experience any unusual movements or muscle twitches, as that could be a sign that the sodium levels are affecting your brain function."

4.3 Check for Fluid Status and Intake/Output
↳ Ensure the patient's fluid intake and output are balanced. An overload of fluids, such as excessive IV fluids, may exacerbate hyponatremia. If indicated, monitor urine output and assess for signs of oedema.

What to say:
↳ "I'll check your fluid intake and urine output to make sure we're not overloading your body with fluids."

Step 5: Management and Post-Procedure Care

5.1 Notify the Medical Team

↪ Report any abnormal findings to the attending physician or the medical team. If the patient shows signs of severe hyponatremia, such as altered mental status or seizure activity, immediate intervention (e.g., sodium correction) may be required.

What to say:

↪ "I've documented all the findings, and I will let the doctor know about your sodium levels and any symptoms you've been having."

5.2 Administer IV Fluids as Ordered

↪ If the physician has ordered IV fluids (e.g., hypertonic saline) to correct sodium levels, prepare and administer them according to protocol. Close monitoring of fluid intake is essential.

What to say:

↪ "I'll be starting an IV fluid infusion now to help balance your sodium levels as ordered by the doctor."

5.3 Provide Comfort and Symptom Relief

↪ Provide any necessary medications to alleviate symptoms such as pain or headache, as prescribed by the physician.

What to say:
- "Let me know if you experience any discomfort, and I'll make sure we address that as well."

Step 6: Documentation and Reporting

6.1 Document the Assessment and Findings
- Record the time and date of the assessment, the patient's sodium levels, GCS score, vital signs, and any symptoms observed. Document all interventions provided and the patient's response.

Example Documentation:
- "Hyponatremia (Na 113) identified in post-op TKR patient Mr. Robert Harris. GCS score 15/15, vital signs stable. Patient reports mild headache, no confusion or seizures observed. Sodium correction initiated with IV fluids as per physician's order. Patient tolerated the procedure well."

6.2 Report Abnormal Findings to Medical Team
- If any significant changes are noted in the patient's condition, especially worsening neurological symptoms or worsening hyponatremia, report to the physician immediately.

What to say:
- "I have documented all findings and reported them to the medical team for further review and management." team in a timely manner.

연습 Scenario 4:
Sore Throat After Holiday Lymph Node Assessment

* Time: 10 minutes
* Setting: Outpatient Clinic
* Situation: Assessment of Sore Throat and Lymph Nodes

✏ Example Scenario Description:

You are a registered nurse in an outpatient clinic. Your patient, Mrs. Emily Carter, a 35-year-old female, presents with complaints of a sore throat after returning from a holiday abroad. She has also noticed some tenderness in her neck. You are tasked with assessing her throat and lymph nodes to identify possible causes, such as an infection (e.g., viral or bacterial pharyngitis, tonsillitis, or a respiratory infection).

✐ Candidate Instructions:

Step 1: Patient Communication and Preparation

1.1 Introduce Yourself and Confirm Identity
↳ Knock on the door, greet the patient, and confirm their identity.

What to say:
↳ "Good morning, Mrs. Carter. My name is [Your Name], and I am your nurse today. Could you please confirm your full name and date of birth? Thank you."

1.2 Explain the Situation and Obtain Consent
↳ Explain the purpose of assessing her sore throat and lymph nodes, and what the process will involve.

What to say:
↳ "I understand you've been experiencing a sore throat and some tenderness in your neck since returning from your holiday. I'll be assessing your throat and checking the lymph nodes around your neck and under your jaw to help determine what may be causing this. It will involve me gently feeling your neck and asking you to open your mouth. Are you comfortable with that?"

: Obtain verbal consent before proceeding.

1.3 Ensure Patient Comfort and Positioning
↳ Make sure the patient is seated comfortably. Have them relax with their head slightly tilted back and their neck exposed for easier examination.

What to say:
- "Please make yourself comfortable and tilt your head slightly back so I can examine your throat and lymph nodes."

Step 2: Assessment of Sore Throat and Lymph Nodes

2.1 Assess the Throat
- Using a tongue depressor, gently open the patient's mouth and inspect the throat for signs of redness, swelling, exudates (pus), or lesions. Also, check for signs of tonsillitis or pharyngitis.

What to say:
- "Please open your mouth wide for me. I'm going to check your throat now. You may feel some pressure, but it shouldn't be painful."

2.2 Palpate the Lymph Nodes
- Gently palpate the lymph nodes in the neck (anterior, posterior, submandibular, and supraclavicular regions) and under the jawline to assess for any tenderness, swelling, or enlargement.

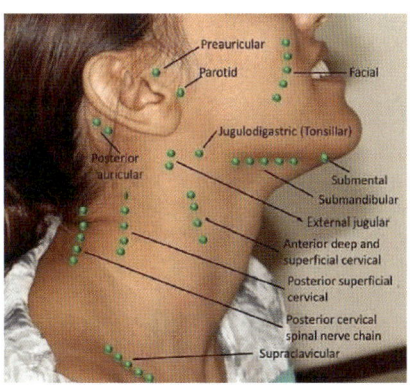

What to say:

→ "I'm now going to check the lymph nodes in your neck and under your jaw. Let me know if you feel any discomfort."

2.3 Assess for Signs of Infection

→ Look for signs of systemic infection such as fever, chills, or fatigue, which can accompany throat infections (bacterial or viral). Take the patient's temperature if they appear febrile.

What to say:

→ "Do you feel feverish, or have you experienced chills recently? Let me know if you feel tired or unwell."

Step 3: Physiological Assessment

3.1 Measure Vital Signs

→ Measure the patient's temperature, heart rate, respiratory rate, and blood pressure. Fever may suggest an infection, and tachycardia may accompany it.

What to say:

→ "I'm going to take your vital signs now, starting with your temperature, to help me understand if there's any infection causing your symptoms."

3.2 Auscultate for Respiratory Signs

→ Listen to the patient's lungs for any abnormal sounds

such as wheezing or crackles, which may suggest a respiratory infection.

What to say:

↳ "I'm going to listen to your lungs now to make sure everything sounds clear and normal."

3.3 Check for Other Symptoms of Infection

↳ Ask about associated symptoms, such as body aches, fatigue, or difficulty swallowing, which can help indicate whether the sore throat is viral or bacterial.

What to say:

↳ "Are you having any difficulty swallowing, or feeling achy or overly tired? These symptoms can sometimes point to a viral or bacterial infection."

Step 4: Post-Procedure Care and Patient Education

4.1 Provide Symptom Relief and Comfort

↳ Advise the patient on how to relieve their symptoms while awaiting further diagnostic results, including drinking fluids, using throat lozenges, or taking over-the-counter pain relievers as needed.

What to say:

↳ "You can try drinking warm fluids or use throat lozenges to help soothe your throat. If the pain worsens or you develop any new symptoms, let us know."

4.2 Monitor for Complications

➣ Educate the patient about signs of complications, such as difficulty breathing, worsening pain, or spreading redness in the throat, which would warrant immediate medical attention.

What to say:

➣ "If you notice any difficulty breathing, worsening pain, or if the redness in your throat spreads, please seek immediate medical attention."

4.3 Advise Follow-Up

➣ Suggest follow-up care if necessary, including seeing a doctor for further evaluation or testing (e.g., throat culture or rapid strep test).

What to say:

➣ "Depending on the findings, you may need further testing, such as a throat culture, to determine whether it's viral or bacterial. If necessary, we will schedule a follow-up."

Step 5: Documentation and Reporting

5.1 Document the Assessment and Findings

➣ Record the time and date of the assessment, symptoms reported by the patient, vital signs, findings from the physical exam (throat inspection and lymph node palpation), and any interventions provided.

Example Documentation:
⤻ "Sore throat assessment performed on patient Mrs. Emily Carter. Throat inspection revealed mild erythema and no exudates. Lymph nodes tender but not enlarged. No fever or difficulty breathing. Vital signs stable. Advised to use throat lozenges and monitor symptoms."

5.2 Report Abnormal Findings
⤻ If any abnormal findings are noted (e.g., significantly swollen lymph nodes, high fever, or difficulty breathing), report these to the physician for further evaluation.

What to say:
⤻ "I've documented the findings and will report any concerning symptoms to the physician for further assessment."

❹ 전문적인 답변

Station Four: Professional Responsibility

---

* Time: 10 minutes
* Setting: General practice clinic
* Patient: Mr. John Smith, 55 years old
* Situation: Medication Administration and Error Reporting

✒ Example Example Scenario Description:

You are a nurse working in a busy medical ward, responsible for administering medications to multiple patients. While preparing to administer a prescribed medication to one of your patients, you accidentally misread the medication order and administer the wrong dose. Upon realizing the mistake, you feel a sense of urgency to ensure the patient's safety and correct the error promptly.

> 당신은 바쁜 병동에서 여러 명의 환자에게 약물을 투여하는 일을 맡고 있는 간호사입니다. 한 환자에게 처방된 약물을 투여하기 위해 준비하던 중, 약물 처방을 잘못 읽고 잘못된 용량을 투여하게 됩니다. 실수를 깨닫자마자 당신은 환자의 안전을 보장하고 오류를 신속하게 수정해야 한다는 촉박감이 듭니다.

✑ Candidate instructions:

1. Acknowledge the Error

As soon as you realize the error, it's important to verbally acknowledge that a mistake has occurred. Be open, honest, and calm when explaining the situation. It's crucial to immediately recognize the mistake, as this sets the tone for the next steps in the process. Be sure to reassure the patient that you're taking the necessary actions to correct it promptly.

> 실수를 깨닫자마자 오류가 발생했음을 인정하는 것이 중요합니다. 상황을 설명할 때는 솔직하고 차분하게 설명해야 합니다. 실수를 즉시 인식하는 것이 중요하며, 이는 이후 절차의 진행 방향을 설정하는 데 큰 역할을 합니다. 환자에게는 필요한 조치를 신속하게 취하고 있음을 확신시켜 주어야 합니다.

What to say:

"I've just realized that I have administered the incorrect dose of your medication. I want to acknowledge this mistake right away and take immediate action to correct it. Your safety is my top priority, and I will make sure everything is handled carefully from here on out."

> "저는 지금 환자분께 잘못된 용량의 약물을 투여했다는 것을 깨달았습니다. 제 실수를 인정하고, 즉각적인 조치를 취하겠습니다. 환자분의 안전이 최우선이며, 앞으로 모든 과정이 신중하게 처리되도록 하겠습니다."

2. Patient Safety

Once you've acknowledged the error, your next priority is the patient's safety. Immediately assess the patient for any signs of adverse reactions or discomfort that may have resulted from the medication error. This includes checking vital signs such as blood pressure, heart rate, oxygen saturation, and respiratory rate. Be alert for any symptoms like shortness of breath, dizziness, or unusual pain. It's essential to monitor the patient closely for any changes and offer reassurance while doing so.

> 오류를 인정한 후, 다음으로 가장 중요한 것은 환자의 안전입니다. 약물 오류로 인해 발생할 수 있는 부작용이나 불편함의 징후를 즉시 사정해야 합니다. 이는 혈압, 심박수, 산소 포화도, 호흡수와 같은 생명징후를 확인하는 것을 포함합니다. 호흡곤란, 어지러움, 또는 이상한 통증과 같은 증상에 주의해야 합니다. 환자의 상태 변화를 면밀히 모니터링하고, 그 과정에서 환자에게 안심을 주는 것이 중요합니다.

What to say:

"I'm going to monitor your condition closely right now. I'll check your blood pressure, heart rate, and breathing to make sure you're not experiencing any adverse reactions. If you feel any discomfort, pain, or notice anything unusual, please let me know immediately."

> "저는 지금 지금부터 당신의 상태를 면밀히 모니터링할 것입니다. 혈압, 심박수, 호흡을 확인하여 부작용이 없으신지 점검하겠습니다. 불편함이나 통증을 느끼거나 이상한 점이 있으면 즉시 말씀해 주세요."

3. Reporting the Error

Following hospital protocol is critical in this situation. As soon as you have realised error, report the error to your supervisor or the appropriate authority within the healthcare system. Make sure you follow the steps outlined in the protocol for medication errors, which typically include documentation and notification of the healthcare team. Ensure that the error is properly recorded in the patient's medical chart, which helps maintain accurate records for both legal and clinical purposes.

> 이 상황에서는 병원 프로토콜을 따르는 것이 매우 중요합니다. 약물오류를 발견하는 순간 오류를 상급자나 의료 시스템 내의 적절한 담당자에게 보고해야 합니다. 약물 오류에 대한 프로토콜에 따라 필요한 절차를 따르도록 합니다. 이는 일반적으로 문서화와 의료 팀에 대한 통지를 포함하며, 환자의 의무기록에 오류가 정확히 기록되도록 해야 합니다. 이는 법적 및 임상적인 목적을 위해 정확한 기록을 유지하는 데 도움이 됩니다.

What to say:

"I will report this medication error to my supervisor immediately. I'll follow the necessary protocol to document the situation correctly, and I'll make sure all relevant information is recorded in your medical record so that we can address this thoroughly."

> "약물 오류를 즉시 제 상사에게 보고하겠습니다. 상황을 정확히 문서화하기 위해 필요한 프로토콜을 따를 것이며, 모든 관련 정보가 귀하의 의무기록에 기록되도록 하여 이 문제를 철저히 해결할 수 있도록 하겠습니다."

4. Communication

Clear and compassionate communication is key when dealing with the patient and their family. Take the time to explain what happened, why it happened, and what steps you are taking to address the situation. Being transparent helps to build trust, and addressing any concerns the patient or family may have is essential. Keep the lines of communication open throughout the process, updating them regularly and offering support. This also includes answering any questions they might have and providing reassurance that their safety is the primary concern.

> 환자와 가족을 대할 때는 명확하고 연민심을 가진 마음으로 의사소통을 하는 것이 중요합니다. 무슨 일이 일어났는지, 왜 일어났는지, 그리고 이를 해결하기 위해 어떤 조치를 취하고 있는지 설명하는 데 시간을 투자해야 합니다. 투명하게 소통하는 것은 신뢰를 쌓는 데 도움이 되며, 환자나 가족이 가질 수 있는 우려를 해결하는 것이 필수적입니다. 이 과정 내내 의사소통의 창을 열어 두고, 정기적으로 업데이트를 제공하며 지원을 아끼지 않아야 합니다. 또한, 그들의 질문에 답하고, 환자의 안전이 최우선임을 확신시켜 주는 것도 포함됩니다.

What to say:

"I apologize for the mistake I made in administering your medication. I understand how this can be concerning. I'm taking immediate steps to ensure your safety, including monitoring you closely for any reactions. If you have any questions or concerns, please don't hesitate to ask. I will keep you updated as we monitor your condition."

> "제가 약물을 투여하는 과정에서 실수를 한 점에 대해 사과드립니다. 이로 인해 걱정이 되실 수 있다는 것을 이해합니다. 환자님의 안전을 보장하기 위해 즉시 조치를 취하고 있으며, 반응을 면밀히 모니터링하고 있습니다. 질문이나 우려 사항이 있으시면 언제든지 말씀해 주세요. 환자님의 상태를 모니터링하면서 계속해서 업데이트를 드리겠습니다."

5. Reflective Practice

After addressing the immediate needs of the patient, take the time to reflect on the error and what led to it. Reflective practice involves understanding the circumstances that contributed to the mistake and considering ways to prevent it from happening again. Identify any factors that may have led to the error, whether it was a distraction, a miscommunication, or a procedural issue. It's important to adopt strategies, such as double-checking medications or seeking guidance when unsure, to prevent future errors. Engage in discussions with colleagues to learn from the situation and improve the overall process.

> 환자에게 필요한 즉각적인 사항들을 해결한 후, 실수와 그 원인에 대해 반성하는 시간을 가지는 것이 중요합니다. 이는 실수가 발생한 상황을 이해하고, 그것이 다시 발생하지 않도록 예방할 방법을 고려하는 과정입니다. 실수를 초래한 요인이 무엇이었는지, 예를 들어 방해 요소, 의사소통의 오류, 또는 절차상의 문제 등을 파악해야 합니다. 향후 오류를 방지하기 위해 약물 투여 전에 이중 확인을 하거나 불확실할 때 동료의 도움을 받는 것과 같은 전략을 세우는 것이 중요합니다. 동료들과 이 상황에 대해 논의하고 배우고, 전반적인 프로세스를 개선하는 데 기여해야 합니다.

What to say:

"I'll be reflecting on this situation to understand what caused the error. I know it's crucial to double-check medication orders and doses, and I will ensure that I always do so in the future. I'll also consider seeking assistance from a colleague when I have any doubts to make sure we maintain the highest standards of care. I'll work on improving my own practice to ensure this doesn't happen again."

"저는 이번 상황에 대해 반성하며 실수가 발생한 원인을 이해하려고 노력할 것입니다. 약물 처방과 용량을 이중 확인하는 것이 매우 중요하다는 것을 알고 있으며, 앞으로 항상 그렇게 하도록 할 것입니다. 또한, 불확실할 때는 동료에게 도움을 요청하여 우리가 최고의 케어 를 제공하고 그를 유지할 수 있도록 하겠습니다. 이번 일이 다시 발생하지 않도록 저의 practice을 개선해 나가겠습니다."

연습 Scenario 1:
Informed Consent

* Time: 10 minutes
* Setting: Surgical Ward
* Patient: Mr. James Wilson, 45 years old
* Presenting Complaint: The patient is unsure about the details of the surgery and expresses confusion and uncertainty.

Example Scenario Description:

You are a registered nurse in a surgical ward, preparing Mr. James Wilson, a 45-year-old male patient, for an upcoming surgical procedure. During the preoperative preparation, Mr. Wilson expresses confusion about the surgery and is unsure of its purpose, benefits, and potential risks. He appears anxious and hesitant, which may delay the procedure or compromise his confidence in the care team. Your task is to address his concerns, clarify any misunderstandings, and ensure he provides informed consent before proceeding.

Candidate Instructions:

1. Introduce Yourself and Establish Rapport:

- Greet the patient warmly and introduce yourself by name and role.
- Create a comfortable and safe environment where the patient feels supported to express their concerns.
- Use open-ended questions to encourage the patient to share their thoughts and feelings about the surgery.
- Example statement:
  - "Good morning, Mr. Wilson. My name is [Your Name], and I'll be your nurse today. I understand you have some concerns about your surgery. I'm here to listen and help clarify any questions or uncertainties you may have."

2. Acknowledge and Validate the Patient's Concerns:

- Listen actively and empathetically as the patient explains their confusion or hesitation.
- Avoid dismissing or minimizing their concerns; instead, validate their feelings to build trust.
- Example response:
  - "It's completely normal to feel uncertain or have questions before surgery. This is a big step, and it's important that you feel comfortable and informed before proceeding."

3. Clarify the Details of the Surgery:

- Use clear and non-technical language to explain the purpose, benefits, and potential risks of the surgery.
- Reinforce key points already provided by the surgeon, ensuring consistency in communication.
- Provide written materials, diagrams, or other visual aids if needed to help the patient better understand.
- Example statement:
  - "The purpose of this surgery is to [state purpose]. It's expected to help by [state benefit]. Like any procedure, there are risks involved, such as [list potential risks], but these have been carefully considered by your care team."

4. Assess Understanding and Encourage Questions:

- Ask the patient to repeat their understanding of the procedure to ensure clarity.
- Invite the patient to ask additional questions or raise concerns.
- Example question:
  - "Could you share with me your understanding of the surgery? That way, I can make sure we're on the same page. Is there anything you'd like me to explain in more detail?"

5. Provide Reassurance and Emotional Support:

↳ Acknowledge the patient's anxiety and provide reassurance about the surgical team's expertise and dedication to their safety and well-being.

↳ Example reassurance:
- "You are in excellent hands. The surgical team has performed this procedure many times and will take every precaution to ensure your safety and comfort."

6. Advocate for the Patient's Right to Informed Consent:

↳ If the patient continues to feel unsure or unable to make an informed decision, inform the surgeon or medical team immediately to allow further discussion.

↳ Ensure that the patient has the time and support needed to make an informed choice without feeling pressured.

7. Document the Conversation:

↳ Record the patient's concerns, the information provided, and their response in the medical record.

↳ Note whether the patient appears comfortable proceeding with the surgery or if further discussions are needed with the surgical team.

연습 Scenario 2:
Ethical Dilemma in Patient Care

* Time: 10 minutes
* Setting: Palliative Care Unit
* Patient: Mr. John Roberts, 68 years old
* Presenting Complaint: A terminally ill patient wishes to discontinue treatment, but their family insists on pursuing as many possible measures to prolong life

Example Scenario Description:

You are a registered nurse in a palliative care unit, providing care to Mr. John Roberts, a 68-year-old patient with advanced-stage cancer. During a private conversation, Mr. Roberts shared with you his wish to discontinue further treatment, explaining that he wants to prioritize comfort and quality of life in his remaining time. However, his family members are adamant that every possible medical intervention be pursued to extend his life. This creates an ethical dilemma involving patient autonomy, family dynamics, and the principles of beneficence and non-maleficence. Your task is to handle this sensitive situation by balancing respect for the patient's wishes with compassionate communication with the family and collaboration with the healthcare team.

Candidate Instructions:

1. Patient-Centered Care:

- Arrange a private conversation with the patient to confirm and clarify their wishes regarding discontinuing treatment.
- Use open-ended questions to fully understand their reasoning, preferences, and values, ensuring that they feel heard and supported.
- Provide reassurance that their decision will be respected and that the focus will be on ensuring their comfort and dignity.
- Example statement:
  - "Mr. Roberts, thank you for sharing your thoughts with me. I want to make sure I fully understand your wishes so that we can prioritize your comfort and dignity in the care we provide. Can you tell me more about what's most important to you right now?"

2. Family Communication:

- Arrange a family meeting in a calm and private setting. Begin by acknowledging their emotions and validating their concerns.

- Compassionately explain the patient's wishes and the importance of respecting autonomy in end-of-life care.
- Educate the family about the goals of palliative care, emphasizing that the focus is on comfort and quality of life rather than prolonging suffering.
- Use empathetic language, such as:
  - "I understand how difficult this is for you as a family. It's clear how much you love and care for Mr. Roberts. He has shared his wish to prioritize comfort over further treatments, and our role as healthcare providers is to honor his choices while supporting all of you through this process."

3. Ethical Framework:

- Ground the discussion in ethical principles:
  - **Autonomy:** Respect the patient's right to make decisions about their own care.
  - **Beneficence:** Act in the patient's best interest to maximize comfort and dignity.
  - **Non-maleficence:** Avoid causing unnecessary suffering through aggressive interventions.
  - **Justice:** Ensure that care is fair and in line with ethical standards.
- Communicate these principles to both the patient and family to provide a clear framework for decision-making.

4. Collaboration:

- Involve the multidisciplinary healthcare team, including the attending physician, palliative care specialists, social workers, and a medical ethics consultant, if necessary, to mediate and provide support.
- Collaborate with the team to create a unified approach that aligns with the patient's wishes while addressing the family's concerns.
- Example action: Suggest a family meeting facilitated by a palliative care consultant to help mediate and explore the emotional and ethical aspects of the situation.

5. Documentation:

- Document all conversations with the patient and family in the medical record, including the patient's stated wishes and reasoning.
- Record the details of family meetings, including their concerns and any agreed-upon care plans.
- Ensure the documentation reflects a clear plan of care that aligns with the patient's autonomy and the ethical considerations discussed.

Key Considerations:

- Show empathy and compassion at all times, understanding that this is an emotional and challenging situation for both the patient and family.
- Remain neutral and professional, avoiding judgment while advocating for the patient's autonomy.
- Use clear and non-technical language to ensure that the patient and family fully understand the situation and the care options available.

연습 Scenario 3:
Professional Boundaries

* Time: 10 minutes
* Setting: Medical Ward
* Patient: Mr. James Carter, 45 years old
* Presenting Complaint: Professional boundaries, social media connection

Example Scenario Description:

You are a registered nurse in a medical ward, providing care to Mr. James Carter, a 45-year-old patient recovering from a mild stroke. During his stay, you have developed a good rapport with him, as he appreciated your attentive care and supportive nature. On the day of his discharge, Mr. Carter asks if you could connect with him on social media, expressing that he values your kindness and would like to stay in touch. While his request appears harmless, it presents a potential ethical challenge regarding professional boundaries. Your task is to handle the situation appropriately, ensuring that you maintain professionalism while respecting the patient's feelings.

✍ Candidate Instructions:

1. Acknowledge the Request:
- ⤳ Begin by thanking the patient for their kind words and expressing gratitude for their trust in you.
- ⤳ Acknowledge that you understand why they may want to stay in touch and appreciate their sentiments.

2. Explain Professional Boundaries:
- ⤳ Clearly and respectfully explain the importance of maintaining professional boundaries in healthcare.
- ⤳ Highlight that these boundaries are essential to protect both the patient and the healthcare professional and to maintain the professional integrity of the therapeutic relationship.
- ⤳ For example, you might say:
  - "I truly appreciate your kind offer and the trust you've placed in me. However, as healthcare professionals, it's important for us to maintain clear boundaries to ensure the therapeutic relationship remains professional and focused on your care."

3. Reassure the Patient:

- Reassure the patient that this decision does not impact the quality of care they have received or will receive in the future.
- Emphasize that maintaining boundaries ensures you can continue to provide the best professional care for all your patients.

4. Offer Alternatives:

- Suggest appropriate ways for the patient to stay connected or seek support if needed.
- For example, refer them to hospital follow-up services, patient support groups, or resources where they can connect with healthcare professionals in a structured and professional setting.
- Highlight any available community or hospital resources that align with their interests or needs.

5. Document the Conversation:

- Record the interaction in the patient's medical record, ensuring that the discussion is documented factually and without judgment.
- Include details about the request, your explanation of professional boundaries, and any alternative resources or suggestions provided to the patient.

6. Reflect and Learn:

➤ After the situation, reflect on the importance of maintaining professional boundaries and how such conversations can uphold the standards of nursing practice.

➤ Consider any additional training or policies within your organization that could help address similar situations in the future.

연습 Scenario 4:
Advocating for a Patient's Cultural Needs

* Time: 10 minutes
* Setting: Post-Operative Ward
* Situation: A patient's cultural dietary requirements were not met

✑ Example Scenario Description:

You are a registered nurse working in a post-operative ward. Mrs. Aroha Te Rangi, a 50-year-old patient of Māori descent, has expressed disappointment and frustration that her cultural dietary needs were not considered in her post-operative meal plan. She feels disrespected and is reluctant to engage with the healthcare team further.

This scenario emphasizes the importance of cultural competence, active listening, and effective problem-solving in ensuring patient-centred care. It also highlights the need for clear communication and advocacy to address cultural needs within a healthcare setting.

Candidate Instructions:

1. Introduce Yourself and Actively Listen

Approach Mrs. Te Rangi with respect and introduce yourself. Use active listening skills to fully understand her concerns. Maintain open body language and show empathy.

What to say:

"Kia ora, Mrs. Te Rangi. My name is [Name], and I'm your nurse today. I understand that there's been an issue with your meal plan. Can you share more about what happened so I can help address this for you?"

2. Apologize and Acknowledge the Oversight

Offer a sincere apology for the mistake and acknowledge the impact it has had on her. Validate her feelings and emphasize the importance of respecting her cultural values.

What to say:

"I want to sincerely apologize for this oversight. I understand how important it is for your cultural values to be respected, especially during your recovery. I can see why this would be upsetting, and I'm here to make sure this is resolved."

3. Reassure and Commit to Action

↪ Reassure Mrs. Te Rangi that her concerns are taken seriously and will be addressed promptly. Explain the steps you will take to rectify the issue.

What to say:

↪ "Your concerns are very important to us. I will work with the dietary team right away to ensure your meals reflect your cultural needs moving forward. Please rest assured that we'll resolve this as soon as possible."

4. Collaborate with the Dietary Team

↪ Contact the dietary services to update the patient's meal plan, ensuring it aligns with her cultural dietary preferences. Confirm the details with Mrs. Te Rangi before finalizing.

What to say to the dietary team:

↪ "We need to adjust Mrs. Te Rangi's meal plan to accommodate her cultural dietary requirements. Can we ensure her meals meet these needs starting with the next one?"

What to say to the patient:

↪ "I've spoken with the dietary team, and they'll prepare meals that meet your cultural needs. Can you confirm any specific preferences or restrictions, so we get it just right?"

5. Escalate to the Supervisor if Necessary

➤ If systemic changes are needed, escalate the issue to your supervisor to prevent similar mistakes in the future.

What to say:

➤ "I'd like to escalate this issue to ensure that our processes for meeting cultural dietary needs are improved across the team. This way, we can avoid similar oversights for other patients."

6. Document the Concerns and Actions Taken

➤ Record Mrs. Te Rangi's concerns in her patient notes, including the steps taken to address them and any follow-up plans.

What to document:

➤ "Patient expressed dissatisfaction with her post-operative meal plan not aligning with her cultural dietary needs. Apologized for the oversight and reassured her that the issue will be resolved. Dietary services were contacted to update meal plan per patient's preferences. Patient verbalized understanding and satisfaction with the plan moving forward."

7. Reflect on Cultural Competency

↠ Reflect on the situation to identify how you and the team can improve cultural awareness and sensitivity in patient care. Consider discussing this case in a team meeting to highlight the importance of cultural competency.

What to say to yourself/team:

↠ "This situation highlights the importance of understanding and respecting diverse cultural needs. We should consider additional training or protocols to ensure all patients feel respected and supported during their care."

❺ 응급상황 관리

Station Five: Emergency management

* Time: 10 minutes
* Setting: Outpatient clinic
* Patient: Mr. John Smith, 55 years old
* Situation: A patient who received an antibiotic injection and is now presenting with severe allergic reactions.(Sudden onset of difficulty breathing, swelling of the face and lips, and a rapid, weak pulse)

✒ Example Example Scenario Description:

You are working as a nurse in an outpatient clinic. A patient, who was recently administered an antibiotic injection, suddenly developed severe allergic symptoms, including difficulty breathing, swelling of the face and lips, and a rapid, weak pulse. The patient is visibly anxious and distressed.

> 당신은 외래 진료소에서 간호사로 일하고 있습니다. 최근 항생제 주사를 맞은 환자가 갑자기 심한 알레르기 증상, 즉 호흡 곤란, 얼굴과 입술의 부기, 빠르고 약한 맥박을 보이며, 환자는 명백히 불안하고 고통스러워 보입니다.

✍ Candidate instructions:

1. Recognize the Signs and Symptoms of Anaphylactic Shock:

What the candidate can say:

➢ To the patient: "I can see that you're having trouble breathing, and your face is swelling. These signs suggest you may be having an allergic reaction to the medication. I'm going to help you right away."

> 환자분, 호흡이 어려워지고 얼굴이 부풀어 오른 것을 보니, 약물에 알레르기 반응을 일으키고 있을 수 있습니다. 지금 바로 도와드리겠습니다.

Rationale:

➢ Anaphylactic shock is a life-threatening allergic reaction that requires immediate intervention. The candidate must recognize the signs and symptoms, which include respiratory distress, swelling of the face and lips, and a rapid, weak pulse. Early identification is critical to initiate the proper course of treatment.

> 아나필락틱 쇼크는 즉각적인 개입이 필요한 생명을 위협하는 알레르기 반응입니다. Candidate는 호흡 곤란, 얼굴과 입술의 부기, 빠르고 약한 맥박을 포함한 징후와 증상을 인지해야 합니다. 조기 식별은 적절한 치료 과정을 시작하는 데 매우 중요합니다.

2. Administer the Appropriate Emergency Medications(e.g., Epinephrine):

What the candidate can say:

⤳ To the patient: "I am going to give you an injection of epinephrine to help reverse this allergic reaction. This will help you breathe more easily and reduce the swelling."

> 알레르기 반응을 역전시키기 위해 에피네프린 주사를 드리겠습니다. 이것이 호흡을 더 쉽게 하고 부기를 줄이는 데 도움이 될 것입니다.

Rationale:

⤳ Epinephrine is the first-line treatment for anaphylactic shock. It works by constricting blood vessels to counteract hypotension, relaxing the muscles around the airways to alleviate breathing difficulty, and reducing swelling. Administering this medication quickly can prevent fatal outcomes.

> 에피네프린은 아나필락틱 쇼크의 1차 치료법입니다. 이 약물은 혈관을 수축시켜 저혈압을 예방하고, 기도 주변의 근육을 이완시켜 호흡 곤란을 완화하며, 부기를 줄이는 역할을 합니다. 이 약물을 빠르게 투여하면 치명적인 결과를 예방할 수 있습니다.

3. Implement Airway Management Techniques:

What the candidate can say:

⤳ To the patient: "I'm going to help you breathe more easily. Try to stay calm. I will support your breathing as we get you the necessary treatment."

> 호흡을 더 쉽게 도와드리겠습니다. 차분하게 유지하세요. 필요한 치료를 받으실 수 있도록 호흡완화를 도와드리겠습니다.

Rationale:

↳ Maintaining a clear airway is crucial in patients experiencing anaphylactic shock, as airway constriction and oedema can impede breathing. Elevating the head of the bed can aid in easier breathing, and supplemental oxygen may be required if the patient's oxygen saturation is low.

> 아나필락틱 쇼크를 경험하는 환자에게는 기도를 유지하는 것이 매우 중요합니다. 기도 수축과 부기가 호흡을 방해할 수 있기 때문입니다. 침대 머리를 높이면 호흡이 더 쉬워질 수 있으며, 환자의 산소 포화도가 낮으면 추가 산소 공급이 필요할 수 있습니다.

4. Monitor Vital Signs and Prepare for Possible Advanced Interventions:

What the candidate can say:

↳ To the patient: "I'm going to monitor your vital signs closely to make sure you're stabilizing, and I'll let the doctor know if we need further intervention."

> 환자분, 저는 환자분이 안정되고 있는지 확인하기 위해 활력징후를 면밀히 모니터링할 것이며, 추가 처치가 필요하면 의사에게 보고하겠습니다.

Rationale:

↳ Monitoring vital signs(heart rate, blood pressure, respiratory rate, oxygen saturation) is essential for assessing the effectiveness of the initial interventions and ensuring that the patient is stabilizing. If the patient's condition worsens, further interventions such as fluid resuscitation, additional epinephrine doses, or intubation may be needed.

활력징후(심박수, 혈압, 호흡수, 산소 포화도)를 모니터링하는 것은 초기 처치의 효과를 평가하고 환자가 안정되고 있는지 확인하는 데 필수적입니다. 환자의 상태가 악화되면, 수액 투여, 추가적인 에피네프린 투여 또는 기관내 삽관과 같은 추가 처치가 필요할 수 있습니다.

5. Communicate with the Healthcare Team for Urgent Support:

What the candidate can say:

↳ To the patient(while communicating with the team): "I've given you epinephrine, and I'm monitoring you closely. I'm also calling the doctor and the emergency team to come in right away, just in case you need further treatment."

저는 에피네프린을 드렸고, 환자분을 면밀히 모니터링하고 있습니다. 또한, 추가 치료가 필요할 경우를 대비해 의사와 응급팀에 연락하고 있습니다.

↳ To the healthcare team: "We have a patient with anaphylactic shock. I've administered epinephrine and am monitoring their vital signs. Could you please assist with further management and any necessary interventions?"

아나필락틱 쇼크를 겪고 있는 환자가 있습니다. 에피네프린을 투여하고 활력징후를 모니터링하고 있습니다. 추가 처치 및 필요한 중재에 대해 도와주실 수 있으신가요?"

Rationale:

↪ Clear and effective communication with the healthcare team is crucial to ensure timely and coordinated care. The candidate must promptly inform the doctor and other relevant team members, such as an emergency response team, so they can intervene as needed.

> 의료팀과의 명확하고 효과적인 소통은 신속하고 협력적인 치료를 보장하는 데 중요합니다. 후보자는 의사와 응급 대응팀과 같은 관련 팀원들에게 즉시 상황을 알리고, 필요시 그들이 개입할 수 있도록 해야 합니다.

6. Document the Incident:

Rationale:

↪ Documentation ensures legal and clinical accountability. The nurse must record the sequence of events, including symptoms, interventions, and any communications with other healthcare professionals. This will be critical for ongoing patient care and potential future legal or clinical reviews.

✳ Example

```
Date/Time: [date and time of the event]
Patient: Mr. [patient name]
DOB: [patient's date of birth]
Location: Outpatient Clinic
```

↪ Subjective:

- Patient presents with complaints of difficulty breathing, facial swelling, and a weak, rapid pulse after receiving an antibiotic injection. The patient appears anxious and visibly distressed.

↪ Objective:

- Vital signs:
    · HR, BP, RR, O2 Sat, Temperature
- Physical Exam Findings:
    · Swelling noted on the face and lips.
    · Respiratory distress observed.
    · Rapid and weak pulse.
    · Patient appears anxious and is struggling to breathe.

↪ Assessment:

- Clinical signs and symptoms consistent with anaphylactic shock following antibiotic administration. Immediate intervention is required to manage the patient's airway, breathing, and circulation.

↪ Plan/Intervention:

1.1 Administered epinephrine 0.5mg IM as per anaphylactic shock protocol.

1.2 Positioned the patient with the head elevated to assist with breathing.
1.3 Administered oxygen via [insert method] at [insert flow rate].
1.4 Vital signs are being monitored every [insert interval] to assess response to treatment.
1.5 Notified the doctor and emergency team regarding the patient's condition for further support.
1.6 Documented patient's response to the interventions and ongoing monitoring.

↠ **Patient Response:**
- After epinephrine injection, patient's respiratory effort slightly improved. Facial swelling continues but is less pronounced. Pulse remains weak but less rapid. Patient reports some relief from breathing difficulty but remains anxious.

↠ **Follow-up/Plan:**
- Continue to monitor vital signs and symptoms closely.
- Emergency team and doctor to reassess patient for possible further treatment.
- Continue to monitor for any signs of deterioration or worsening condition.

Signature:

[nurse's name and title]

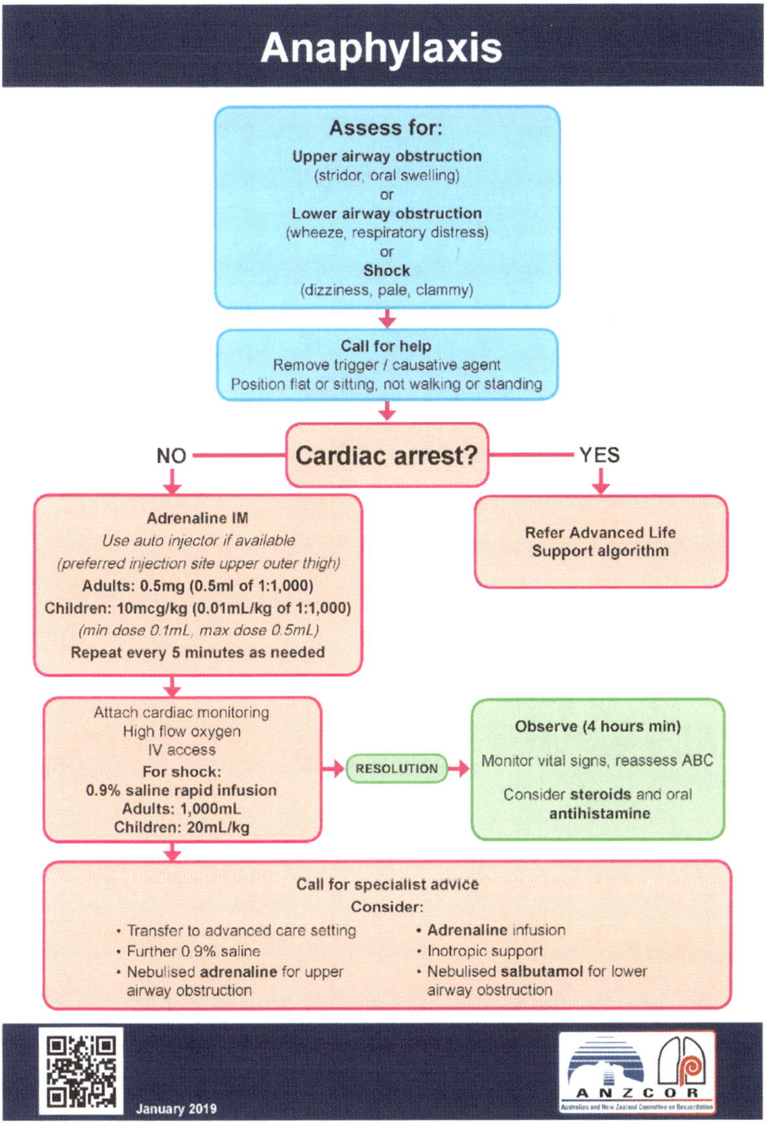

Anaphylaxis

Assess for:
Upper airway obstruction
(stridor, oral swelling)
or
Lower airway obstruction
(wheeze, respiratory distress)
or
Shock
(dizziness, pale, clammy)

↓

Call for help
Remove trigger / causative agent
Position flat or sitting, not walking or standing

↓

Cardiac arrest?

NO → **Adrenaline IM**
Use auto injector if available
(preferred injection site upper outer thigh)
Adults: 0.5mg (0.5ml of 1:1,000)
Children: 10mcg/kg (0.01mL/kg of 1:1,000)
(min dose 0.1mL, max dose 0.5mL)
Repeat every 5 minutes as needed

YES → **Refer Advanced Life Support algorithm**

↓

Attach cardiac monitoring
High flow oxygen
IV access
For shock:
0.9% saline rapid infusion
Adults: 1,000mL
Children: 20mL/kg

→ RESOLUTION → **Observe (4 hours min)**
Monitor vital signs, reassess ABC
Consider **steroids** and oral **antihistamine**

↓

Call for specialist advice
Consider:
- Transfer to advanced care setting
- Further 0.9% saline
- Nebulised **adrenaline** for upper airway obstruction
- **Adrenaline** infusion
- Inotropic support
- Nebulised **salbutamol** for lower airway obstruction

January 2019

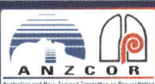
ANZCOR
Australian and New Zealand Committee on Resuscitation

연습 Scenario 1:
Severe Asthma Attack

* Time: 10 minutes
* Setting: Outpatient Clinic
* Patient: 45-year-old female
* Presenting Complaint: Severe shortness of breath, wheezing, and cyanosis

Example Scenario Description:

A 45-year-old female patient with a known history of asthma arrives at the outpatient clinic in severe respiratory distress. She is experiencing shortness of breath, audible wheezing, and cyanosis, which are clear signs of a severe asthma attack. The patient appears anxious and is struggling to speak in full sentences due to difficulty breathing. Immediate intervention is required to stabilize her condition, prevent further deterioration, and provide life-saving care.

This scenario requires the candidate to rapidly assess the patient's respiratory status, administer appropriate medications, and monitor the patient closely while preparing for potential advanced airway management if her condition worsens. Effective communication with the healthcare team and accurate documentation are essential.

✍ Candidate Instructions:

1. Perform a Rapid Assessment of Respiratory Status:

- Observe the patient for signs of respiratory distress, such as the use of accessory muscles and inability to speak in full sentences.
- Assess respiratory rate, effort, and lung sounds(e.g., wheezing).
- Check oxygen saturation levels and vital signs, including heart rate and blood pressure.

What to say:

- To the patient: "I see you're having difficulty breathing. I'm going to check your oxygen levels and listen to your lungs to see what's going on."

2. Administer Prescribed Bronchodilators and Corticosteroids:

- Administer a short-acting bronchodilator(e.g., salbutamol) via a nebulizer or metered-dose inhaler with a spacer.
- If prescribed, administer corticosteroids(e.g., prednisone) to reduce airway inflammation.

What to say:

↬ To the patient: "I'm going to give you medication through this nebulizer to help open your airways. It should make it easier for you to breathe."

3. Monitor Oxygen Saturation and Provide Supplemental Oxygen:

↬ Continuously monitor oxygen saturation using a pulse oximeter.
↬ Provide supplemental oxygen via a mask or nasal cannula to maintain saturation levels above 94%.

What to say:

↬ To the patient: "I'm going to place this oxygen mask on you to help increase the oxygen levels in your blood. Please try to breathe as slowly and deeply as you can."

4. Prepare and Assist with Potential Advanced Airway Management:

↬ Be ready to assist with intubation or other advanced airway techniques if the patient's condition worsens.
↬ Gather necessary equipment, such as an airway kit, and alert the resuscitation or critical care team.

What to say:

↳ To the healthcare team: "The patient's condition is critical, and I'm preparing airway equipment in case advanced intervention is needed. Please stand by to assist if necessary."

5. Communicate with the Healthcare Team and Document the Care Provided:

↳ Notify the physician and other team members about the patient's condition and interventions performed.

↳ Document the patient's symptoms, vital signs, medications administered, and response to treatment in the medical record.

What to say:

↳ To the healthcare team: "We have a patient experiencing a severe asthma attack. I've administered salbutamol and supplemental oxygen, and her oxygen saturation is now at 92%. She remains in distress, so we may need to consider additional interventions."

↳ To the patient: "I've informed the doctor about your condition, and we're working as a team to ensure you get the best care."

연습 Scenario 2:
Hypoglycaemic Emergency

* Time: 10 minutes
* Setting: Medical ward, patient's Room
* Patient: 58-year-old male
* Presenting Complaint: Unconscious with symptoms of severe hypoglycaemia

Example Scenario Description:

A 58-year-old male patient with a history of diabetes is found unconscious in his room. Initial observation indicates symptoms consistent with severe hypoglycaemia, such as cold, clammy skin and unresponsiveness. Immediate intervention is required to stabilize the patient, prevent further complications, and ensure their safety.

This scenario requires the candidate to act quickly by confirming hypoglycaemia, administering appropriate treatment, and closely monitoring the patient's response. Effective communication with the healthcare team and accurate documentation of the incident are critical components of the task.

✈ Candidate Instructions:

1. Perform a Rapid Blood Glucose Test to Confirm Hypoglycaemia:

↠ Use a glucometer to check the patient's blood sugar level.

↠ Identify whether the blood glucose level is critically low(e.g., below 4 mmol/L).

What to say:

↠ To yourself : "This patient's symptoms are consistent with severe hypoglycaemia. I need to confirm their blood glucose level immediately."

↠ To the patient(if semi-conscious): "I'm going to check your blood sugar to see what's causing this."

2. Administer an Appropriate Treatment:

↠ If the patient is conscious but unable to swallow effectively, administer glucose gel buccally.

↠ If unconscious or unable to take oral glucose, administer intravenous dextrose or intramuscular glucagon, as per hospital protocol.

What to say:

↠ To the patient(if semi-conscious): "Your blood sugar is very low. I'm going to give you some glucose to raise it and help you feel better."

- To the healthcare team: "The patient is unresponsive, and their blood sugar is critically low at 2.3 mmol/L. I'm administering IV dextrose immediately."

3. Monitor the Patient's Vital Signs and Level of Consciousness:

- Continuously monitor vital signs(blood pressure, heart rate, respiratory rate, and oxygen saturation).
- Reassess blood glucose levels after treatment to confirm improvement.
- Watch for signs of recovery, such as improved consciousness and responsiveness.

What to say:
- To yourself: "I need to monitor the patient's vital signs closely to ensure they're stabilizing after treatment."
- To the patient(if regaining consciousness): "Your blood sugar is coming up, and you should start to feel better soon. I'll keep monitoring you closely."

4. Prepare to Manage Possible Complications and Ensure Patient Safety:

- Be ready to address potential complications, such as seizures or prolonged unresponsiveness.
- Place the patient in a safe position(e.g., lateral recovery position) to prevent aspiration if unconscious.

What to say:

↳ To the healthcare team: "The patient is improving, but I'm preparing for possible complications, such as a seizure or further loss of consciousness."

↳ To the patient(if conscious): "You're in a safe position now, and we're closely monitoring you to prevent any further complications."

5. Communicate with the Healthcare Team and Document the Incident:

↳ Notify the attending physician and other relevant team members of the patient's condition, interventions performed, and response to treatment.

↳ Document the event, including the initial assessment, blood glucose levels, medications administered, and patient response, in the medical record.

What to say:

↳ To the healthcare team: "The patient was unresponsive due to severe hypoglycaemia, with a blood sugar level of 2.3 mmol/L. I've administered IV dextrose, and their level of consciousness is improving. I'll document the interventions and continue to monitor."

↳ To the patient(if conscious): "The doctor has been informed of your condition, and we're taking all the necessary steps to ensure your safety and recovery."

연습 Scenario 3:
Acute Myocardial Infarction(Heart Attack)

* Time: 10 minutes
* Setting: Emergency Department
* Patient: 58-year-old male
* Presenting Complaint: Chest pain, shortness of breath, and diaphoresis

Example Scenario Description:

A 58-year-old male presents to the emergency department with complaints of severe chest pain radiating to the left arm, shortness of breath, and excessive sweating(diaphoresis). These symptoms are indicative of a potential acute myocardial infarction(heart attack). Immediate intervention is required to stabilize the patient, reduce the risk of further cardiac damage, and prepare for advanced interventions if needed.

This scenario emphasizes the candidate's ability to perform a rapid assessment, administer emergency medications, and effectively communicate with the healthcare team. Prompt and accurate documentation of care is essential to ensure continuity of care.

✒ Candidate Instructions:

1. Perform a Rapid Assessment, Including Obtaining a History and Vital Signs:

- Assess the patient's symptoms, such as the location, intensity, and duration of chest pain.
- Obtain vital signs, including blood pressure, heart rate, respiratory rate, and oxygen saturation.
- Check for additional symptoms, such as nausea or dizziness, and inquire about the patient's medical history(e.g., previous heart issues, medications, allergies).

What to say:
- To the patient: "I see you're experiencing chest pain and shortness of breath. I'm going to ask you some questions and check your vital signs to determine what's happening."
- Internally: "These symptoms strongly suggest a myocardial infarction. I need to act quickly to stabilize the patient."

2. Administer Prescribed Medications, Such as Aspirin and Nitro-glycerine:

- Administer aspirin(chewed, if prescribed) to reduce blood clot formation.

- Administer nitro-glycerine(GTN stray, Sublingually- if prescribed) to relieve chest pain by improving blood flow to the heart.
- Monitor the patient's blood pressure before and after administering nitro-glycerine to ensure stability.

What to say:

- To the patient: "I'm going to give you aspirin to thin your blood and GTN spray to help relieve your chest pain. Let me know if you feel any relief or if the pain worsens."
- To the healthcare team: "The patient has taken aspirin and given 2 puffs of GTN spray. I'll monitor for any changes in blood pressure or pain levels."

3. Prepare and Assist with Electrocardiogram(ECG) Monitoring:

- Set up the ECG machine and attach leads to the patient's chest as per protocol.
- Obtain a 12-lead ECG to confirm the diagnosis and identify the type of myocardial infarction.
- Report ECG findings promptly to the physician or healthcare team.

What to say:

- To the patient: "I'm going to place some electrodes on your chest to monitor your heart's electrical activity. This will help us better understand what's happening."
- To the healthcare team: "The ECG shows ST-elevation consistent with myocardial infarction. I'm notifying the cardiology team immediately."

4. Monitor the Patient's Condition and Be Prepared for Advanced Cardiac Life Support(ACLS) If Needed:

- Continuously monitor the patient's vital signs and cardiac rhythm.
- Be prepared to initiate ACLS protocols, including defibrillation or advanced airway management, if the patient's condition deteriorates.
- Ensure emergency resuscitation equipment is readily available.

What to say:

- To the patient: "We're keeping a close eye on your heart and vital signs to ensure you're stable. Please let me know if you feel worse or have new symptoms."
- To the healthcare team: "The patient's vital signs are stable, but I'm preparing for potential ACLS intervention if needed."

5. Communicate with the Healthcare Team and Document All Care Provided:

- Update the attending physician and cardiology team on the patient's condition and interventions performed.
- Document all assessments, medications administered, ECG results, and any changes in the patient's condition.

What to say:

- To the healthcare team: "The patient presented with chest pain and diaphoresis. Aspirin and GTN were administered, and the ECG confirmed ST-elevation myocardial infarction. Vital signs are being closely monitored, and the patient is stable for now. I'll continue to document the care provided."
- To the patient: "We've informed the cardiology team and are preparing for further treatment. You're in good hands, and we'll keep you updated on the next steps."

연습 Scenario 4:
Seizure management

- **Time**: 10 minutes
- **Setting**: General Ward
- **Patient**: 28-year-old male
- **Presenting Complaint**: Active seizure witnessed by staff

✎ Example Scenario Description:

A 28-year-old male admitted for observation after a recent head injury suddenly began to have a tonic-clonic seizure. The patient exhibits jerking movements, is unresponsive, and has laboured breathing during the episode. Immediate intervention is required to ensure the patient's safety, prevent complications, and manage the seizure effectively.

This scenario emphasizes the nurse's ability to identify the type of seizure, provide first-line management, and collaborate with the healthcare team for further interventions. Accurate documentation of the event is also crucial for ongoing care.

✒ Candidate Instructions:

1. Ensure the Patient's Safety:

- Clear the area of any objects that could cause harm during the seizure.
- Position the patient on their side to maintain an open airway and prevent aspiration.
- Protect the patient's head with a soft object, such as a folded towel or pillow.

What to say:

- To yourself: "The patient is having a tonic-clonic seizure. My priority is to keep them safe and ensure their airway is clear."
- To the patient(after the seizure ends): "You've had a seizure, but you're safe now. I'm here to help you."
- To others: "Please move back to give the patient space. I need someone to time the seizure and inform the medical team."

2. Monitor the Seizure:

- Note the time the seizure started and observe its duration.
- Observe the characteristics of the seizure, such as limb movements, facial expressions, and any vocalizations.
- Identify any post-seizure confusion or lingering symptoms once the seizure ends.

What to say:

↬ To the healthcare team: "The seizure started at 10:15 AM and lasted approximately two minutes. The patient exhibited tonic-clonic movements and is now regaining consciousness."

3. Administer Emergency Medications If Prescribed:

↬ If the seizure lasts longer than 5 minutes or repeats without full recovery, administer prescribed medications such as IV lorazepam or rectal diazepam.
↬ Ensure all interventions are performed under aseptic conditions and as per hospital protocol.

What to say:

↬ To the patient(if conscious): "I'm going to administer medication to help stop the seizure. It will help you feel better."
↬ To the healthcare team: "The patient's seizure lasted over five minutes. I've administered lorazepam as prescribed."

4. Monitor the Patient Post-Seizure(Postictal Phase):

↬ Check vital signs, including heart rate, blood pressure, and oxygen saturation.
↬ Assess the patient's level of consciousness and orientation.
↬ Provide reassurance and ensure the patient is comfortable while recovering.

What to say:

- To the patient: "You're recovering from a seizure. I'm going to check your vital signs to make sure everything is okay."
- To the healthcare team: "The patient is in the postictal phase, with stable vital signs but some confusion. Monitoring will continue."

5. Communicate with the Healthcare Team and Document the Incident:

- Inform the attending physician about the seizure and the interventions performed.
- Document the time, duration, and characteristics of the seizure, as well as any medications administered and the patient's response.

What to say:

- To the healthcare team: "The patient experienced a two-minute tonic-clonic seizure. Interventions included maintaining safety, positioning, and administering lorazepam. Vital signs are stable post-seizure."
- To the patient: "I've informed the doctor about your seizure. We'll monitor you closely and discuss any further treatment you may need.

❻ 임상 술기(상처드레싱 교환)

Clinical Skills

- **Time**: 10 minutes
- **Setting**: Medical Ward
- **Situation**: Indwelling Catheter Insertion(IDC) for Urinary Retention.

✎ Example Example Scenario Description:

You are a registered nurse working in a medical ward. Your patient, Mr. James Anderson, a 72-year-old male, has been experiencing acute urinary retention secondary to benign prostatic hyperplasia(BPH). He has a distended bladder, complains of severe lower abdominal discomfort, and has not passed urine in over eight hours despite hydration. His doctor has ordered an indwelling urinary catheter(IDC) to relieve the retention. Your task is to explain the procedure to the patient, prepare for catheterization, insert the catheter safely using aseptic technique, ensure proper aftercare, and document the procedure appropriately.

당신은 Medical병동에서 근무하는 간호사입니다. 담당 환자, James Anderson씨(72세 남성)는 양성 전립선 비대증(BPH)으로 인한 급성 배뇨 정체를 경험하고 있습니다. 그는 방광 팽만감을 느끼고 심한 하복부 불편감을 호소하며, 수분 보충에도 불구하고 8시간 이상 소변을 보지 못했습니다. 그의 의사는 배뇨 정체를 해소하기 위해 도뇨관(IDC)을 삽입하도록 지시하였습니다. Candidate로써 당신은 환자에게 시술 절차를 설명하고, 도뇨관 삽입을 위한 준비를 하며, 무균 기술을 사용하여 도뇨관을 안전하게 삽입하고, 적절한 시술 후 관리 및 기록을 작성하는 것입니다.

Candidate Instructions:

Step 1: Patient Communication and Preparation

1.1. Knock on the door, introduce yourself, and confirm patient identity.

➢ "Hello Mr. Anderson, my name is [Your Name], and I am your nurse today. Can you confirm your full name and date of birth for me?"

> 노크를 하고, 자신을 소개한 후 환자의 신원을 확인합니다.
> "안녕하세요, Anderson 씨. 제 이름은 [본인의 이름]이고, 오늘 당신을 돌볼 간호사입니다. 성함과 생년월일을 확인해 주실 수 있나요?"

1.2. Explain the procedure in simple terms.

➢ "I understand you have been experiencing some discomfort due to difficulty passing urine. The doctor has prescribed an indwelling urinary catheter, which is a small flexible tube that will be inserted into your bladder to help drain the urine. This will relieve the pressure and discomfort you are feeling. The procedure should only take a few minutes, and I will ensure it is as comfortable as possible for you. Do you have any concerns or questions before we begin?"

절차를 간단한 용어로 설명합니다.
"소변을 보는데 어려움이 있어 불편함을 겪고 계신 것을 이해합니다. 의사 선생님께서 도뇨관을 삽입하라고 처방하셨습니다. 도뇨관은 작은 유연한 튜브로, 이를 방광에 삽입하여 소변을 배출하는 데 도움을 줄 것입니다. 이렇게 하면 현재 느끼고 계신 압박감과 불편함을 해소할 수 있습니다. 시술은 몇 분 정도만 소요되며, 최대한 편안하게 진행되도록 하겠습니다. 시술을 시작하기 전에 궁금한 점이나 걱정되는 사항이 있으신가요?"

1.3. Obtain informed consent.

↳ "If you're happy for us to proceed, I will begin preparing the equipment and ensure everything is done with sterile technique to prevent infection."

동의서를 받습니다. (Organisation에 따라서 Written 이나 Verbal로 받으면 됩니다, 뉴질랜드에서는 특별한 Written consent가 필요하지는 않고 환자 챠트에 기록해주면 됩니다)
"진행해도 괜찮으시다면, 장비를 준비하고 감염 예방을 위해 모든 절차가 무균 기술로 진행되도록 하겠습니다."

1.4. Ensure privacy and comfort.

↳ Close the curtain and door.

↳ Assist the patient into a supine position with legs slightly apart.

↳ Cover the patient with a drape, exposing only the necessary area.

개인 정보 보호 및 편안함을 보장합니다.
- 커튼과 문을 닫습니다.
- 환자가 무릎을 약간 벌린 상태로 평평한 자세가 되도록 도와줍니다.
- 필요한 부위만 노출되도록 커버로 환자를 덮습니다.

Step 2: Equipment Preparation & Aseptic Technique

2.1. Gather equipment:

- ↪ Catheter insertion kit(including sterile gloves, drapes, antiseptic solution, lubricating gel, forceps, and catheter)
- ↪ Indwelling catheter of appropriate size(usually 14-16Fr for males, 12-14Fr for females)
- ↪ Sterile water for balloon inflation(usually 10ml)
- ↪ Urine collection bag
- ↪ PPE(gloves, gown, and mask if required)

> **장비 준비:**
> - 도뇨관 삽입 키트(무균 장갑, 덮개, 소독액, 윤활 젤, 겸자, 도뇨관 포함)
> - 적절한 크기의 도뇨관(남성의 경우 보통 14-16Fr, 여성의 경우 12-14Fr)
> - 풍선 팽창을 위한 무균 생리식염수(보통 10ml)
> - 소변 수집 백
> - PPE(장갑, 가운, 필요 시 마스크)

2.2. Perform hand hygiene and put on PPE.

- ↪ Open the catheterization kit using sterile technique.
- ↪ Wear sterile gloves and maintain aseptic technique throughout.

> **손 위생을 수행하고 PPE를 착용합니다.**
> - 도뇨관 삽입 키트를 무균 기술로 엽니다.
> - 무균 장갑을 착용하고 시술 내내 무균 기술을 유지합니다.

2.3. Perineal Cleansing and Preparation

↳ Male patient:
- Retract the foreskin(if uncircumcised) and hold the penis at a 90-degree angle.
- Cleanse the meatus with antiseptic solution from the urethral opening outward in a circular motion.
- Apply sterile lubricating gel to the catheter tip.

↳ Female patient:
- Separate the labia using non-dominant hand.
- Cleanse the urethral opening with antiseptic from top to bottom(front to back).
- Apply sterile lubricating gel to the catheter tip.

회음 부위 세정 및 준비
- 남성 환자(** 남성환자의 IDC insertion의 경우 뉴질랜드에서는 추가로 트레이닝을 받은후 Procedure를 진행할수 있습니다)
  · 포경 수술을 하지 않은 경우, 음경을 90도 각도로 들어 foreskin을 뒤로 젖힌다.
  · 소독액을 사용하여 요도구를 원을 그리며 요도 개구부에서 바깥쪽으로 세정한다.
  · 도뇨관 끝에 무균 윤활 젤을 바른다.
- 여성 환자:
  · 주로 쓰지 않는 손으로 음순을 벌린다.
  · 소독액을 사용하여 요도 개구부를 위에서 아래로(앞에서 뒤로) 세정한다.
  · 도뇨관 끝에 무균 윤활 젤을 바른다.

Step 3: Catheter Insertion and Urine Drainage

3.1. Insert the catheter using a steady motion:

↳ "Mr. Anderson, you may feel some pressure or slight discomfort as I insert the catheter. Take slow, deep breaths to help relax."
- Insert the catheter until urine flows into the tube.

- Advance the catheter 2-3 cm further to ensure it is correctly positioned.

> **도뇨관을 일정한 움직임으로 삽입합니다:**
> "Anderson 씨, 도뇨관을 삽입하면서 압박감이나 약간의 불편함을 느끼실 수 있습니다. 천천히 깊게 숨을 쉬며 이완을 도와주세요."
> - 도뇨관을 삽입하여 소변이 튜브로 흐르도록 합니다.
> - 도뇨관을 2-3cm 더 밀어넣어 정확한 위치에 있는지 확인합니다.

↬ "I can see the urine flowing now. I'm just advancing the catheter a little more to ensure it's in the correct position."
  - Inflate the catheter balloon with sterile water to secure placement.
  - Gently pull back slightly until resistance is felt.
↬ "The catheter is now secured in place. I will attach it to the drainage bag, and you should start to feel relief soon."

> "이제 소변이 흐르는 것을 볼 수 있습니다. 도뇨관을 조금 더 밀어넣어 정확히 위치시킬게요."
> - 도뇨관 풍선에 무균 생리식염수로 공기를 넣어 위치를 고정시킵니다.
> - 저항을 느낄 때까지 살짝 뒤로 당깁니다.
> "도뇨관이 이제 고정되었습니다. 배액 백에 연결할 것이며, 곧 불편함이 완화될 것입니다."

Step 4: Post-Insertion Care and Patient Education

4.1. Secure the catheter and ensure proper positioning

- Attach the drainage bag to the bed below bladder level.
- Secure the catheter to the patient's thigh to prevent movement.
- Ensure no kinks or obstructions in the tubing.

> **도뇨관을 고정하고 적절한 위치를 확인합니다.**
> - 배액 백을 방광보다 낮은 침대에 연결합니다.
> - 도뇨관을 환자의 허벅지에 고정하여 움직이지 않도록 합니다.
> - 튜브에 꼬이거나 막힌 부분이 없는지 확인합니다.

4.2. Assess patient response

- "How are you feeling now, Mr. Anderson? The discomfort should start to subside as your bladder empties."
- Monitor urine output, color, and consistency.
- Observe for signs of infection or complications(e.g., bleeding, pain, leakage).

> **환자의 반응을 평가합니다.**
> "지금 기분이 어떠신가요, Anderson 씨? 방광이 비어가면서 불편함이 점차 줄어들 거예요."
> - 소변의 양, 색상 및 일관성을 모니터링합니다.
> - 감염이나 합병증의 징후(예: 출혈, 통증, 누수 등)를 관찰합니다.

4.3. Provide patient education

→ "This catheter will remain in place as per the doctor's orders. It is important to keep the drainage bag below the bladder level to ensure proper drainage. If you feel any discomfort, pain, or notice cloudy or foul-smelling urine, please let the nursing team know immediately. I will check on you regularly and make sure everything is working properly."

> **환자 교육을 제공합니다.**
> "이 도뇨관은 의사의 지시에 따라 계속 유지됩니다. 적절한 배액을 위해 배액 백을 방광보다 낮은 위치에 두는 것이 중요합니다. 불편함, 통증을 느끼거나 소변이 흐릿하거나 악취가 나면 즉시 간호팀에 알려주세요. 저는 정기적으로 확인하고 모든 것이 제대로 작동하는지 확인하겠습니다."

Step 5: Documentation and Reporting

→ Record the time and date of catheter insertion.
→ Note the catheter size, type, and amount of balloon inflation.
→ Document the patient's response and urine output.
→ Report any abnormal findings to the doctor.

> **문서화 및 보고**
> - 도뇨관 삽입 시간과 날짜를 기록합니다.
> - 도뇨관 크기, 유형 및 풍선 팽창 양을 기재합니다.
> - 환자의 반응과 소변 양을 문서화합니다.
> - 비정상적인 소견이 있으면 의사에게 보고합니다.

✳ Study Tips!!

- Practice catheter insertion on mannequins to perfect technique.
- Memorize the step-by-step process to ensure efficiency during timed OSCE exams.
- Familiarize yourself with different catheter types and sizes for male and female patients.
- Understand catheter-related complications(e.g., infections, trauma, blockages) and how to manage them.
- Use ISBAR when escalating concerns about catheterization difficulties.
- Time yourself during practice to ensure completion within the OSCE time limit.

Fig 1. **Inserting a catheter into a female patient**

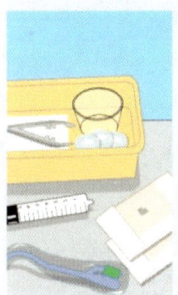

1a. After risk assessment prepare the patient and the equipment

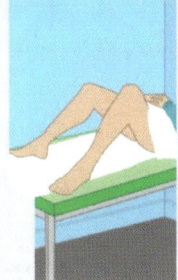

1b. Assist the patient into a supine position with knees bent and feet apart

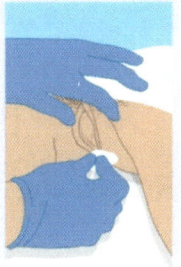

1c. Clean the labia with 0.9% sodium chloride to reduce infection risk

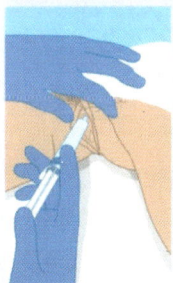

1d. Instill anesthetic or lubricating gel into the urethra to reduce pain and/or urethral trauma

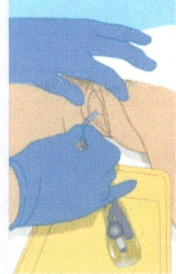

1e. Hold the labia open and insert the catheter into the bladder using your dominant hand

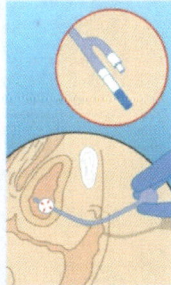

1f. Inflate the balloon and connect to a drainage device or catheter valve

〈Female IDC insertion 예시〉

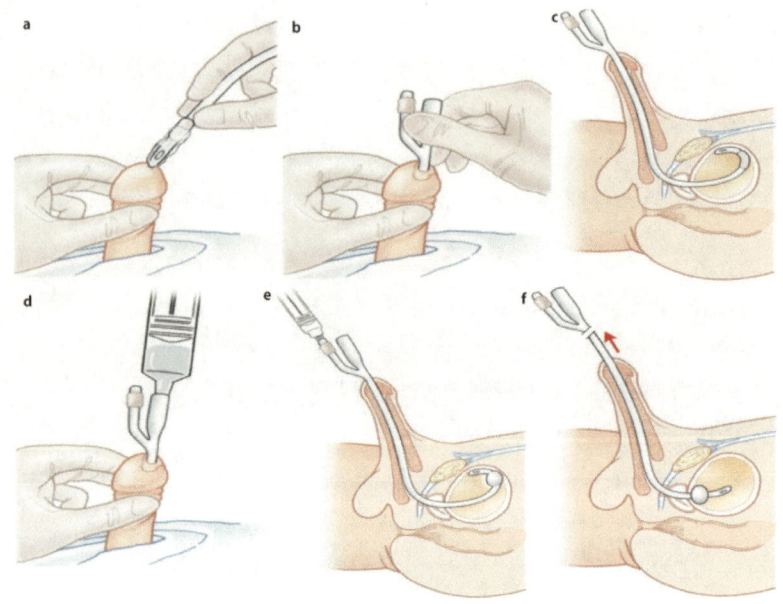

〈Male IDC insertion 예시〉

연습 Scenario 1:
Nasogastric tube Insertion

* Time: 10 minutes
* Setting: Medical Stroke Ward
* Situation: Nasogastric tube Insertion

Example Example Scenario Description:

You are a registered nurse working in a medical Stroke ward. Your patient, Mrs. Emily Roberts, a 65-year-old female, has been unable to take oral nutrition due to dysphagia following a recent stroke. The doctor has prescribed nasogastric tube(NGT) insertion for enteral feeding.

Your task is to explain the procedure, safely insert the nasogastric tube using correct technique, confirm its placement, and document the procedure.

⚐ Candidate Instructions:

Step 1: Patient Communication and Preparation

1.1 Introduce Yourself and Confirm Identity
↝ Knock on the door, greet the patient, and check their identity.

What to say:
↝ "Good morning, Mrs. Roberts. My name is [Your Name], and I am your nurse today. Could you please confirm your full name and date of birth? Thank you."

1.2 Explain the Procedure and Obtain Consent
↝ Provide a clear explanation of the procedure and its purpose.

What to say:
↝ "Your doctor has recommended that we insert a small, flexible tube through your nose and into your stomach. This will help provide you with essential nutrition and fluids since you have difficulty swallowing. The procedure might be slightly uncomfortable, but I will guide you through it and make sure you are as comfortable as possible. Do you have any questions or concerns before we proceed?"

: Obtain verbal consent before proceeding.

1.3 Ensure Patient Comfort and Positioning

- Sit the patient upright(at least 45-90 degrees) to reduce the risk of aspiration.
- Provide tissues in case of discomfort(e.g., nasal irritation or gagging).

What to say:

- "I will have you sit up nice and straight to help the tube pass more easily. If you feel any discomfort, take slow breaths through your mouth. If needed, we can pause at any time."

Step 2: Equipment Preparation & Aseptic Technique

2.1 Gather Required Equipment

- Nasogastric tube(appropriate size, typically 12-16Fr)
  : Check the tube size and expiry date before use.
- Lubricating gel(water-soluble)
- 50 mL syringe(for aspiration and flushing)
- Glass of water with a straw(if patient can swallow)
- pH indicator strips(to confirm placement)
- Adhesive dressing or fixation tape
- PPE(gloves, apron, and mask if necessary)
- Disposable kidney dish and tissues

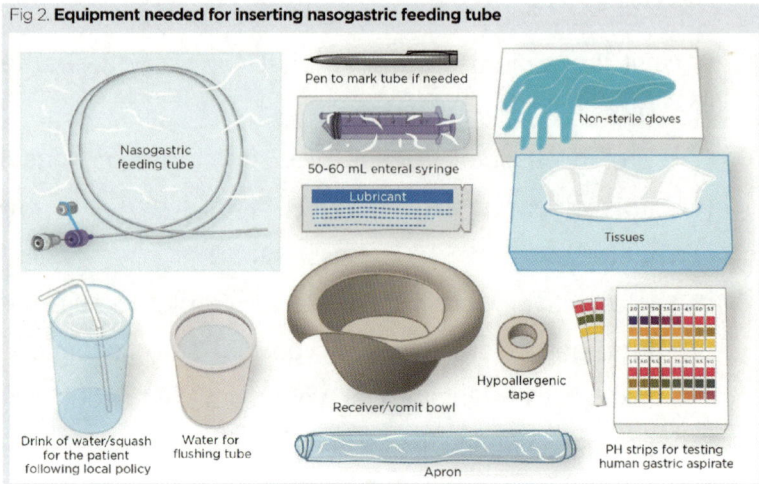

Fig 2. **Equipment needed for inserting nasogastric feeding tube**

2.2 Perform Hand Hygiene and Wear PPE

↳ Wash hands thoroughly and wear non-sterile gloves.

↳ Apply water-soluble lubricant to the first 10-15 cm of the tube.

What to say:

↳ "I am now preparing your tube with some lubricant to help it pass more smoothly."

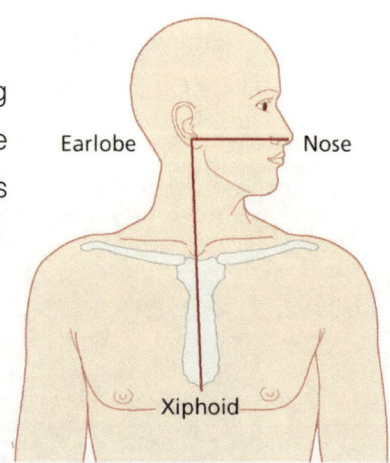

Step 3: Nasogastric Tube Insertion

3.1 Measure and Mark the Tube Length

- Measure from the tip of the nose → earlobe → xiphoid process(stomach).
- Mark the measurement with tape or a marker.

What to say:

- "To ensure the tube reaches your stomach, I will measure it from your nose to your earlobe and then down to your stomach area."

3.2 Insert the Tube Gently and Safely

- Ask the patient if they have any nose surgery or injury history of the of nose and avoid on that side
- Ask the patient to tilt their head slightly forward(chin to chest) to assist passage into the oesophagus.
- Advance the tube gently along the nostril floor toward the back of the throat.

What to say:

- "I will now gently insert the tube through your nose. You might feel a tickling sensation, and your eyes may water a little—this is normal. Please take slow, deep breaths through your mouth."
- If the patient gags or coughs excessively, stop and allow them to recover before continuing.
- Encourage swallowing as the tube advances(offer sips of water via straw if safe to do so).

What to say:

↪ "Please take small sips of water and swallow as I advance the tube. This will help guide it into your stomach."

↪ Advance the tube until it reaches the marked position.

Step 4: Confirm Placement

4.1 Methods to Confirm Tube Placement

↪ Aspirate gastric contents using a syringe and check the pH.

↪ pH should be ≤5.5, indicating correct gastric placement.

↪ DO NOT use auscultation(air insufflation) to confirm placement, as it is unreliable.(Not recommended as the best practice now)

What to say:

↪ "I will now check the tube placement by drawing out some stomach contents and testing the pH."

↪ If pH is too high(>6), the tube may be misplaced(e.g., in the lungs)—STOP and seek medical review.

↪ If safe placement is confirmed, secure the tube with adhesive tape to the nose.

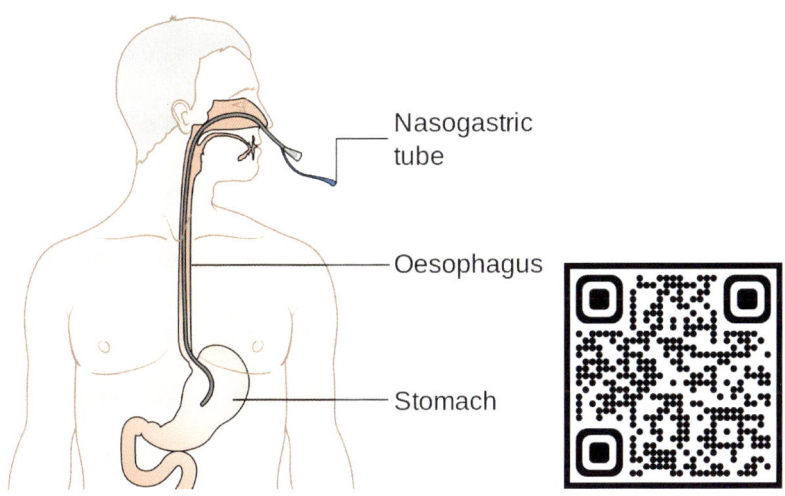

Step 5: Post-Insertion Care and Patient Education

5.1 Secure the Tube and Attach to the Feeding System

↳ Secure the tube to the nose and ensure it is not pulling on the patient's nostrils.

↳ Attach the tube to the prescribed feeding system or connect to free drainage if for decompression.

What to say:

↳ "The tube is now in place, and I have secured it. I will attach it to the feeding system shortly."

5.2 Monitor for Complications

↳ Observe for coughing, respiratory distress, pain, or discomfort.

↳ Check for leakage or kinking of the tube.

↳ Monitor for nausea, bloating, or aspiration signs.

What to say:

➻ "If you feel any nausea, discomfort, or difficulty breathing, please let me know immediately."

Step 6: Documentation and Reporting

➻ Record the time and date of insertion.
➻ Document the size and type of NGT used.
➻ Record the pH confirmation result and method used.
➻ Note any patient response or complications.
➻ Report any abnormal findings to the medical team.

Example Documentation:

➻ "Inserted a 14Fr nasogastric tube via right nostril. Tube length measured and marked appropriately. Placement confirmed with aspirate pH of 5.0. Secured with adhesive tape. Patient tolerated the procedure well, with no immediate complications. Will monitor for tolerance and signs of aspiration."

연습 Scenario 2:
Changing a Colostomy Bag

* Time: 10 minutes
* Setting: General Surgical Ward
* Situation: Changing a Colostomy Bag

✒ Example Example Scenario Description:

You are a registered nurse working in a General Surgical ward. Your patient, Mr. John Harrison, a 58-year-old male, has had a colostomy for the past 1 week following a bowel surgery. He requires assistance in changing and cleaning his colostomy bag. Your task is to explain the procedure, safely remove and replace the colostomy bag using correct technique, and provide patient education

✒ Candidate Instructions:

Step 1: Patient Communication and Preparation

1.1 Introduce Yourself and Confirm Identity
- Knock on the door, greet the patient, and check their identity.

What to say:
- "Good morning, Mr. Harrison. My name is [Your Name], and I am your nurse today. Could you please confirm your full name and date of birth? Thank you."

1.2 Explain the Procedure and Obtain Consent
- Provide a clear explanation of the procedure and its purpose.

What to say:
- "Today, I will assist you in changing and cleaning your colostomy bag. This process helps maintain hygiene and ensures the bag is secure and comfortable. If you feel any discomfort, please let me know immediately. Do you have any questions or concerns before we start?"
  : Obtain verbal consent before proceeding.

1.3 Ensure Patient Comfort and Positioning
- Position the patient in a comfortable, seated, or supine position with good privacy.

What to say:
- "I'll make sure you're comfortable and ensure your privacy throughout this process. If you feel any discomfort, let me know, and I can make adjustments."

Step 2: Equipment Preparation & Aseptic Technique

2.1 Gather Required Equipment

- Colostomy bag(appropriate size and type)
- Scissors(if needed to trim the flange)
- Disposable gloves
- Moist wipes or warm water with soap for cleaning
- Adhesive remover(if necessary)
- Skin barrier wipes or paste
- Disposal bag for the used colostomy bag and contents
- Tissues or gauze
- Colostomy bag clips or closure device
- Barrier film spray(if required)

2.2 Perform Hand Hygiene and Wear PPE

- Wash hands thoroughly and put on disposable gloves.

What to say:

- "I am now putting on gloves and preparing everything needed to change the colostomy bag."

Step 3: Removing the Old Colostomy Bag

3.1 Position and Expose the Colostomy

- Ensure the patient is positioned comfortably and expose the colostomy site while maintaining privacy.

What to say:

- "I'm now going to remove your old colostomy bag. Let me know if you experience any discomfort or pain during this process."

3.2 Remove the Old Colostomy Bag
- Gently peel the adhesive away from the skin, starting from one edge and slowly working around the bag to minimize discomfort.
- If necessary, use an adhesive remover to help loosen the adhesive without causing skin irritation.

What to say:
- "I'm going to remove the bag slowly to avoid any irritation to the skin. You may feel some mild pulling or discomfort as I do this."

3.3 Dispose of the Old Bag and Contents
- Dispose of the old bag and contents in a sealed waste bag.

Step 4: Cleaning and Skin Care

4.1 Clean the Stoma and Surrounding Skin
- Use warm water and a mild soap or pre-moistened wipes to gently clean around the stoma and the surrounding skin.
- Dry the area gently with tissues or gauze.

What to say:
- "I'm cleaning the stoma area now to ensure it's hygienic. Please let me know if you feel any discomfort or irritation."

4.2 Check the Stoma for Signs of Infection

⤻ Inspect the stoma for any signs of infection(redness, swelling, discharge).

⤻ Check the surrounding skin for irritation or breakdown.

What to say:

⤻ "I'm checking the skin around your stoma to make sure everything is healthy and healing properly. Let me know if you notice any pain or changes in the area."

Step 5: Preparing and Applying the New Colostomy Bag

5.1 Prepare the New Colostomy Bag

⤻ Cut the new colostomy bag flange to the appropriate size, ensuring it fits snugly around the stoma without being too tight.

What to say:

⤻ "I'm preparing the new bag and adjusting it to fit your stoma comfortably."

5.2 Apply the New Colostomy Bag

⤻ Peel off the adhesive backing of the bag and gently place it over the stoma.

⤻ Press the adhesive flange against the skin to ensure a secure seal.

⤻ Ensure the bag is firmly attached, with no leaks or gaps.

What to say:

↠ "I'm now placing the new bag over your stoma, ensuring it is snug and secure."

5.3 Secure the Bag and Attach Closure Device

↠ Attach the bag to the closure device(clip or similar) and ensure it is properly sealed.

What to say:

↠ "The bag is now in place, and I'm ensuring it's securely sealed."

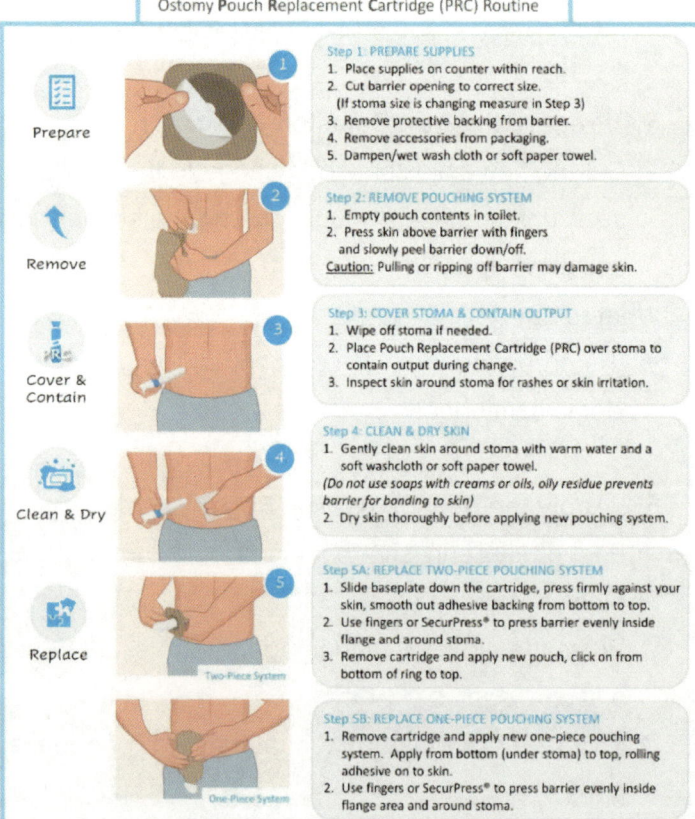

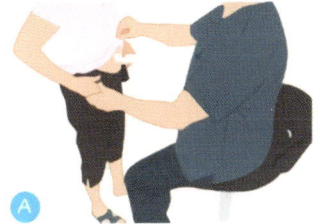
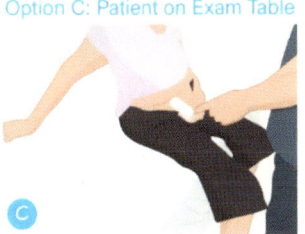
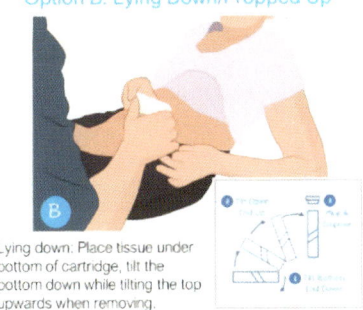

Lying down: Place tissue under bottom of cartridge, tilt the bottom down while tilting the top upwards when removing.

Step 6: Post-Procedure Care and Patient Education

6.1 Check the Colostomy Bag for Comfort and Leaks

- Ensure the patient feels comfortable and the bag is securely attached without any leaks.

What to say:

- "Please let me know if you feel any discomfort or if the bag feels like it's pulling or leaking."

6.2 Educate the Patient on Care and Maintenance

- Guide caring for the colostomy bag, including when to change it, signs of complications, and proper hygiene.

What to say:

⤳ "Be sure to check the bag regularly for leaks, and change it when needed, typically every 2-3 days. Keep the skin around your stoma clean and dry. If you notice any signs of infection or skin irritation, please let me know."

Step 7: Documentation and Reporting

⤳ Record the time and date of the colostomy bag change.
⤳ Document the appearance of the stoma and surrounding skin, any signs of infection or irritation, and any patient concerns.
⤳ Report any abnormalities(e.g., stoma infection, skin breakdown) to the healthcare team.

Example Documentation:

⤳ "Changed colostomy bag for Mr. Harrison, with appropriate bag size and secure fit. Stoma clean with no signs of infection or irritation. Patient tolerated procedure well and was educated on self-care. Will monitor for any signs of leakage or infection."

✴ Study Tips!!

- Practice changing colostomy bags on mannequins or in simulation settings.
- Familiarize yourself with different types of colostomy bags and how to adjust them for individual needs.
- Learn how to assess and manage stoma complications(infection, skin irritation, etc.).
- Time yourself during practice to ensure efficiency and comfort in performing the procedure.

연습 Scenario 3:
Monitoring Blood Glucose Levels(BGLs)

* Time: 10 minutes
* Setting: Medical Ward
* Situation: Monitoring Blood Glucose Levels(BGLs)

Example Example Scenario Description:

You are a registered nurse working in a medical ward. Your patient, Mrs. Sarah Thompson, a 72-year-old female, has been diagnosed with type 2 diabetes and requires regular monitoring of her blood glucose levels(BGLs). You are tasked with explaining the procedure to her, accurately measuring her BGL, and providing necessary education on the results. Your task is to explain the procedure, safely check the patient's blood glucose, interpret the results, and document the procedure.

✍ Candidate Instructions:

Step 1: Patient Communication and Preparation

1.1 Introduce Yourself and Confirm Identity

➢ Knock on the door, greet the patient, and check their identity.

What to say:

➢ "Good morning, Mrs. Thompson. My name is [Your Name], and I am your nurse today. Could you please confirm your full name and date of birth? Thank you."

1.2 Explain the Procedure and Obtain Consent

➢ Provide a clear explanation of the procedure and its purpose.

What to say:

➢ "I'm going to check your blood glucose levels today. This test will give us an idea of how well your body is managing sugar levels. It's a simple test where I will take a small drop of blood from your finger. You might feel a tiny prick, but it won't take long. Do you have any questions or concerns before we start?"

: Obtain verbal consent before proceeding.

1.3 Ensure Patient Comfort and Positioning

➢ Ensure the patient is comfortable and has their hand clean and accessible. Position the patient with their hand at heart level.

What to say:

⤳ "Please rest your hand on your lap and make sure it's relaxed. We'll get started shortly."

Step 2: Equipment Preparation

2.1 Gather Required Equipment

⤳ Blood glucose meter(appropriate brand/model)
⤳ Test strips for the glucose meter
⤳ Lancet device and lancet needles
⤳ Alcohol swabs or antiseptic wipes
⤳ Tissues or gauze
⤳ Gloves
⤳ Sharps container for disposal

: Ensure all equipment is in working order and properly stored.

2.2 Perform Hand Hygiene and Wear PPE

⤳ Wash hands thoroughly and put on gloves.

What to say:

⤳ "I'm washing my hands now and putting on gloves to ensure everything is clean before I test your blood glucose levels."

Step 3: Blood Glucose Measurement

3.1 Prepare the Blood Glucose Meter and Test Strip

⤳ Insert the test strip into the blood glucose meter, ensuring it is ready to receive the blood sample.

What to say:
- "I'm preparing the test strip and getting the glucose meter ready for the reading."

3.2 Prepare the Lancet Device
- Set the lancet device to the appropriate depth for the patient's skin type.
- Gently massage the patient's hand or ask them to make a fist to encourage blood flow.

What to say:
- "I'm getting the lancet device ready and will prepare your finger for the test."

3.3 Clean the Finger Site
- Clean the patient's fingertip with an alcohol wipe and allow it to dry to avoid interfering with the test result.

What to say:
- "I'm now cleaning your finger to make sure it's hygienic before I take the sample."

3.4 Prick the Finger and Obtain Blood Sample
- Choose the side of the fingertip(not the center) and use the lancet device to obtain a small drop of blood.
- Ensure the lancet is used only once and discarded into the sharp's container immediately.

What to say:
- "I'm going to prick your finger now. You may feel a tiny sting."

연습 Scenario 4:
Central Venous Catheter Dressing Method

* **Time**: 10 minutes
* **Setting**: Surgical Ward
* **Situation**: Central Venous Catheter Dressing Method

Example Example Scenario Description:

You are a registered nurse working in a surgical ward. Your patient, Mr. James Reynolds, a 58-year-old male, has a central venous catheter(CVC) in place for long term antibiotics administration. The catheter needs a dressing change, and checked for signs of infection, patency, and any other complications. Your task is to safely change the dressing, check the catheter port, and ensure proper aseptic technique during the procedure.

3.5 Apply Blood to Test Strip
- Touch the blood drop to the test strip in the glucose meter.

What to say:
- "Now, I'm applying the blood to the test strip. It will only take a few seconds to get the result."

Step 4: Interpretation of Results and Patient Education

4.1 Interpret the Blood Glucose Reading
- Wait for the result to appear on the blood glucose meter screen.
- Identify whether the BGL is within the normal range(typically 4-7 mmol/L before meals, and less than 10 mmol/L after meals—values may vary based on patient condition).

What to say:
- "Your current blood glucose level is [result] mmol/L. Based on the result; we will discuss any necessary steps to manage your blood sugar levels."

4.2 Provide Patient Education on the Results
- Educate the patient on what the results mean in simple terms(e.g., whether it is too high, too low, or within a healthy range) and any immediate actions to take.
- Discuss the importance of managing blood glucose and how it affects their overall health.

What to say:
- "Your blood glucose level is [result]. If it's within the normal range, that's great! If it's too high or low, I will let you know how we should proceed. Maintaining healthy blood glucose levels is important for preventing complications from diabetes. Regular monitoring can help manage your condition effectively."

4.3 Provide Recommendations
- If the blood glucose level is outside the normal range, offer appropriate guidance(e.g., eating a snack, administering insulin, or calling the doctor).

What to say:
- "If your blood glucose is too high/low, I will recommend that we take the necessary steps, like adjusting your medication or having a snack, as per the doctor's orders."

Step 5: Post-Procedure Care and Documentation

5.1 Dispose of Used Equipment Properly
- Safely dispose of the lancet in the sharps container and any other waste in the appropriate bin.

What to say:
- "I'm disposing of the lancet and other used materials now."

5.2 Record the BGL Measurement and Any Action
- Document the blood glucose level, time of the t any actions or recommendations mad adjustments to insulin or diet).

Example Documentation:
- "Blood glucose level measured at 10:30 AM. Re mmol/L. Patient instructed on proper monitoring and managing blood sugar le immediate action required."

5.3 Provide Reassurance and Offer Further Ass
- Offer reassurance and answer any ques patient may have regarding their blood gluc or the procedure.

What to say:
- "You did great! If you have any more que concerns, feel free to ask. I'm here to anything related to your diabetes managemen

Study Tips!!
- Practice using the blood glucose meter and lancet devices to ens familiarity with the equipment.
- Memorize normal blood glucose ranges and understand how to res abnormal readings.
- Familiarize yourself with the patient's treatment plan, including administration, to ensure proper follow-up actions are provided.
- Time yourself during practice to ensure you are efficient and co during the procedure.

Candidate Instructions:

Step 1: Patient Communication and Preparation

1.1 Introduce Yourself and Confirm Identity

↝ Knock on the door, greet the patient, and check their identity.

What to say:

↝ "Good morning, Mr. Reynolds. My name is [Your Name], and I am your nurse today. Could you please confirm your full name and date of birth? Thank you."

1.2 Explain the Procedure and Obtain Consent

↝ Explain the purpose of the dressing change, what you will do, and why it is important.

What to say:

↝ "I'm going to change the dressing on your central venous catheter today. This will help prevent infection and keep your catheter clean. You may feel some pressure during the procedure, but it shouldn't be painful. Do you have any questions or concerns before we begin?"

: Obtain verbal consent before proceeding.

1.3 Ensure Patient Comfort and Positioning

↝ Ensure the patient is comfortably positioned with the catheter site accessible. If necessary, place a pillow or support to elevate their arm.

What to say:
- "Please lie back or sit in a comfortable position where I can easily access your catheter port."

Step 2: Equipment Preparation and Aseptic Technique

2.1 Gather Required Equipment
- Sterile dressing change kit
- Sterile gloves
- Antiseptic wipes(e.g., chlorhexidine) and stick
- Sterile gauze pads
- Sterile saline solution
- Transparent dressing(e.g., Tegaderm)
- Adhesive tape
- Sterile cotton balls or swabs
- Sharps container for disposal
- Biohazard bag(for used materials)
    : Ensure all equipment is sterile and in good condition.

2.2 Perform Hand Hygiene and Wear PPE
- Wash hands thoroughly and wear sterile gloves.
- If required, wear a mask and apron as additional precautions.

What to say:
- "I'm now washing my hands and wearing gloves to ensure the procedure is as sterile as possible."

Step 3: Central Venous Catheter Port Inspection and Dressing Change

3.1 Inspect the Catheter Port

↳ Before removing the old dressing, carefully inspect the catheter port for any signs of infection, such as redness, swelling, discharge, or warmth. Check the catheter for any kinks or signs of displacement.

What to say:

↳ "I'm just going to inspect the port and surrounding area to ensure everything is in good condition."

3.2 Remove the Old Dressing

↳ Carefully remove the old dressing, ensuring no contamination of the catheter or site. Dispose of it immediately in the appropriate waste container.

What to say:

↳ "I'll now remove the old dressing carefully, ensuring everything stays sterile."

3.3 Clean the Catheter Site

↳ Use an antiseptic wipe or stick(chlorhexidine or alcohol, depending on the protocol) to clean the catheter site. Clean the area in a circular motion starting from the center and moving outward. Allow the area to dry completely.

What to say:

↳ "I'm cleaning the area with antiseptic to prevent any infection."

3.4 Inspect the Catheter for Patency

- Check that the catheter is patent(free of blockage or clotting) by ensuring it is properly secured and in place. Check for any blood return or aspiration if applicable.

What to say:

- "I'm checking the catheter to ensure it is clear and in good working condition. There's no issue with its flow or placement."

Step 4: Apply New Dressing

4.1 Apply a Sterile Dressing

- Apply a new sterile dressing over the catheter site, ensuring the catheter is well-covered and the dressing is securely adhered to the skin. Ensure there are no wrinkles or air bubbles.

What to say:

- "I'm now applying a fresh sterile dressing to protect the catheter and keep the site clean."

4.2 Secure the Dressing

- Use sterile tape to secure the dressing, ensuring it is well-fitted but not too tight to cause discomfort or restrict circulation.

What to say:

- "The dressing is now secure. I'll ensure it's held in place properly so that it stays clean and protected."

Device, Dressing, Tape Strip Removal Instructions
Minimize catheter manipulation during removal.

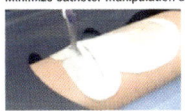
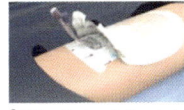
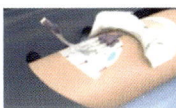
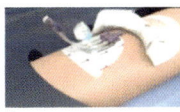

1 Lift catheter lumens, exposing the notches of the perforated tape strip. Gently pull apart the perforated tape strip.

2 Lift the catheter lumen(s) with one hand and place gloved index finger on the base of the device. Utilizing the low and slow removal technique, slowly start removing the tape strips and dressing, as one layer, toward the insertion site.

3 When the catheter hub is exposed, move your gloved finger to secure the catheter hub and continue to remove the dressing until the device is uncovered. Leave the remainder of the dressing in place over the catheter insertion site. Avoid skin trauma by peeling the dressing back, rather than pulling it up from the skin.

4 Remove the device tape strip from the catheter lumen(s).

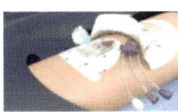
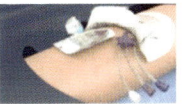
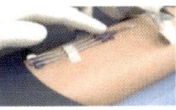

5 Use a gloved finger to stabilize the catheter hub and gently remove the catheter lumen(s) out from under the plastic arm of the device.

6 Secure the catheter with one hand and use your other hand to remove the device from the patient's skin.

7 Stabilize catheter with a sterile tape strip or a gloved finger and carefully remove the remainder of the dressing over the insertion site using the low and slow removal technique.

Step 5: Post-Procedure Care and Patient Education

5.1 Dispose of Used Equipment Properly

↳ Dispose of used materials(e.g., gloves, swabs, old dressing) into the appropriate containers(sharps container, biohazard bag).

What to say:

↳ "I'm disposing of all used materials in the appropriate containers now."

5.2 Monitor for Signs of Complications

↳ Instruct the patient to report any signs of infection, such as increased redness, swelling, pain, or discharge from the catheter site.

What to say:

↳ "Please let me know if you notice any increased pain, redness, swelling, or discharge from the catheter site. These could be signs of infection."

5.3 Provide Patient Education on Care of the Catheter
↠ Educate the patient on how to care for the catheter site at home, including the importance of keeping the site clean and dry and when to seek medical attention.

What to say:
↠ "Make sure to keep the catheter site clean and dry and cover with plastic or wrapping paper. If the dressing becomes wet or lose, you should change it or contact us to arrange for a new one. If you experience any discomfort or see anything unusual around the site, please get in touch immediately."

Step 6: Documentation and Reporting

6.1 Document the Procedure and Patient Response
↠ Record the time and date of the dressing change. Document the condition of the catheter site(any signs of infection, patency of catheter). Note the type of dressing used and any complications or patient response.

Example Documentation:
↠ "Dressed central venous catheter port for patient Mr. James Reynolds. Site inspected for infection, no signs of redness or discharge. Catheter patent. Fresh sterile dressing applied. Patient tolerated the procedure well, no complications noted."

6.2 Report Any Abnormal Findings

↠ If any issues were found with the catheter(e.g., signs of infection, clotting, displacement), report these to the medical team immediately.

What to say:

↠ "I have documented the dressing change and the condition of the catheter. I will report any unusual findings to the medical team for further assessment.

✱ Study Tips!!

- Practice changing dressings on mannequins or with a clinical educator.
- Familiarize yourself with the specific protocol for CVC care in your clinical setting.
- Memorize the key steps for inspecting and maintaining a CVC port.
- Practice effective communication, especially in reassuring patients and educating them post-procedure.
- Time yourself during practice to ensure efficiency during the procedure.

COMPARISON CHART OF WHERE DIFFERENT CENTRAL LINES ARE PLACED

CVC and PICC are used for rapid infusions, long-term medication administration (antibiotics, chemotherapy), total parenteral nutrition and frequent blood draws. Both can be seen in the inpatient and outpatient setting.

LEARNING TIP:

CVC and PICC deliver medications and sample blood from large veins near the heart. These lines end in either the superior vena cava or the right atrium of the heart.

Peripherally Inserted Central Catheters (PICC)

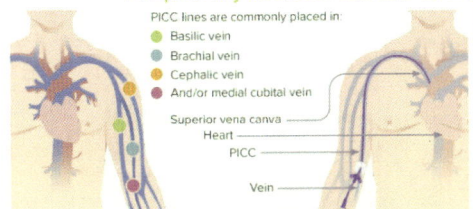

PICC lines are commonly placed in:
- Basilic vein
- Brachial vein
- Cephalic vein
- And/or medial cubital vein

Superior vena canva
Heart
PICC
Vein

LEARNING TIP:

PICC are placed peripherally (ex. arms) but terminate centrally.
There are also midline catheters, which are shorter lines that are also placed peripherally. It is important to note what type of line and where it is placed to determine approved use of medications, fluids, blood draws taken or given from the line.

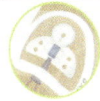

In the outpatient setting, PICC should be covered and protected to prevent dislodging of the catheter and risk of infection.

CLINICAL TIP:

PICC are usually recommended for short to medium term use (4 weeks–6 months), indicated for critically ill and oncology patients.

❼ 약물 투약

Station Seven: Medication Administration

* Time: 10 minutes
* Setting: Medical Ward
* Situation: A patient is scheduled to receive an oral antihypertensive medication, but the nurse must calculate the correct dose based on the doctor's prescription and the medication available.

✐ Example Example Scenario Description:

You are a registered nurse on a medical ward. Mr. John Doe, a 58-year-old patient with hypertension, is scheduled to receive his oral antihypertensive medication. The doctor's prescription specifies 25 mg, but the medication available is in 50 mg tablets, requiring dose calculation.

> 당신은 내과병동에서 근무하는 간호사 입니다. 58세의 고혈압 환자인 John Doe씨가 항고혈압 경구약을 복용할 예정인데요, 의사의 처방은 25mg이지만 병동에 있는 약은 50mg정제로 되어 있어 용량 계산이 필요합니다.

✏ Candidate Instructions:

Your task is to ensure the correct dose is administered by performing accurate calculations, confirming the patient's identity, and monitoring for any adverse reactions post-administration. This scenario tests your competency in medication calculation, safe administration, and patient-centered care.

> Candidate의 task 는 정확한 용량을 계산하고 환자의 신원을 확인하며, 약물을 안전하게 투여하고, 투여후 이상 반응을 모니터링 하는 것입니다. 이 시나리오는 약물 계산 능력, 안전한 약물 관리, 환자 중심의 간호능력을 평가합니다.

1. Verify the Medication Order and Patient Identity

➣ Cross-check the doctor's prescription with the medication available. Use the "7 Rights" of medication administration: right patient, right drug, right dose, right route, right purpose and right time, right documentation. Confirm the patient's identity using at least two identifiers.

> 의사의 처방과 제공된 약물을 교차 확인합니다. 약물 투여의 "7 Rights"을 확인하세요: "올바른 환자, 약물, 용량, 경로, 시간, 목적 기록". 환자의 신원을 확인할때는 적어도 두개의 확인 가능한 identity를 체크합니다.

What to say:

➣ "Good morning, Mr. Doe. My name is [Name], and I'm your nurse today. Can you please confirm your full name and date of birth for me? Thank you. I see you're scheduled to take your blood pressure medication now, and I'll verify the prescription and calculate your dose before we proceed."

좋은 아침입니다, Mr. Doe. 저는 오늘 당신의 간호사 [이름]입니다. 성함과 생년월일을 확인해 주시겠어요? 감사합니다. 오늘 혈압 약을 복용할 예정이고, 처방을 확인한 후 정확한 용량을 계산하겠습니다.

2. Perform Dose Calculation

↳ Calculate the correct dose based on the prescription and available tablets:
  - Doctor's order: 25 mg.
  - Tablet strength: 50 mg per tablet.
  - Required dose = ½ tablet

  처방된 용량과 제공된 정제를 기반으로 정확한 용량을 계산합니다.
↳ 의사의 처방: 25mg.
↳ 정제 용량: 50mg/정.
↳ 필요한 용량 = 0.5 정

What to say(thinking out loud):
↳ "The prescription is for 25 mg, and the tablets are 50 mg each. That means I'll need to give half a tablet to ensure the correct dose."

처방된 용량은 25mg이고, 정제는 50mg입니다. 따라서 정확한 용량을 위해 반 정제를 두어해야 합니다.

3. Explain the Procedure to the Patient and Obtain Consent

↳ Inform the patient about the medication, its purpose, and any potential side effects. Obtain verbal consent before administering.

약물의 목적과 잠재적 부작용에 대해 환자에게 설명합니다. 투여 전에 구두 동의를 얻습니다.

What to say:

➤ "Mr. Doe, your medication is a blood pressure tablet that helps manage hypertension. Today, your dose is 25 mg, which I've calculated to be half a tablet. This medication might occasionally cause dizziness, so please let me know if you feel unwell after taking it. Are you ok to take it?"

Mr. Doe, 이 약물은 혈압을 조절하기 위한 약입니다. 오늘의 용량은 25mg이며, 이를 위해 반 정제를 복용해야 합니다. 이 약물은 가끔 어지럼증을 유발할 수 있으니, 복용 후 불편함을 느끼시면 꼭 알려주세요. 복용 괜찮으시겠어요?"

4. Perform Hand Hygiene and Prepare the Medication

➤ Wash your hands thoroughly, prepare the medication in a clean and safe environment, and ensure accuracy in dose preparation.

손을 철저히 씻고 깨끗하고 안전한 환경에서 약물을 준비합니다.

What to say(while preparing):

➤ "I'm preparing your dose now, ensuring it's accurate. I'll bring it to you shortly."

지금 약을 준비하고 있습니다. 용량이 정확한지 확인 후 바로 가져다 드리겠습니다.

5. Administer the Medication and Monitor the Patient

➤ Provide the medication to the patient and ensure they take it. Observe the patient for any immediate adverse reactions and monitor their blood pressure afterwards.

환자에게 약물을 제공하고 복용을 확인합니다. 즉각적인 이상 반응을 관찰하고 혈압을 포함한 상태를 모니터링합니다.

What to say:

↝ "Here's your medication, Mr. Doe. Please take it with a sip of water. Please let me know if you feel anything unusual.

여기 약이 있습니다, Mr. Doe. 물 한 모금과 함께 드세요. 이상증상이 있으면 바로 알려주세요.

6. Document the Administration

↝ Record the medication administration in the patient's chart, including the dose, time, and any observations.

약물 투여를 포함한 기록을 환자 차트에 정확히 작성합니다.

What to document:

↝ Administered 25 mg of [Medication Name] orally as prescribed. Patient tolerated the medication well, with no immediate adverse reactions noted. Blood pressure and other vitals will be monitored as per protocol.

처방대로 25mg의 [약물 이름]을 경구 투여함. 환자는 약물을 잘 복용하였으며 즉각적인 부작용은 나타나지 않음. 프로토콜에 따라 혈압 및 기타 활력징후를 모니터링할 예정.

연습 Scenario 1:
Transdermal Patch Application

* Time: 10 minutes
* Setting: Medical Ward
* Situation: A patient requires the application of a Fentanyl transdermal patch for chronic pain management, requiring proper assessment, preparation, and education.

✎ Example Scenario Description:

You are a nurse working in a medical ward. Mrs Patel, a 62-year-old patient, has been prescribed a Fentanyl patch for chronic pain management. The patch needs to be applied to a clean, dry, and hairless area of the skin, and the patient must be educated on its use and potential side effects. This scenario assesses your skills in transdermal patch application, patient communication, and education.

Candidate Instructions:

1. Verify Medication Order and Check Patient Identity

Confirm the doctor's order for the Fentanyl patch and ensure the correct medication and dose. Verify the patient's identity using two identifiers(e.g., name and date of birth).

What to say:

"Good morning, Mrs. Patel. My name is [Your Name], and I'll be assisting with your pain management today. May I confirm your name and date of birth? Thank you. I'll be applying a Fentanyl patch to help with your chronic pain. Let me explain the process and answer any questions you might have."

2. Explain the Procedure and Obtain Consent

Discuss the purpose of the patch, how it works, and what the patient can expect. Obtain verbal consent before proceeding.

What to say:

"This patch is designed to provide continuous pain relief over the next few days. It's applied to your skin and will slowly release the medication into your bloodstream. You may notice some mild side effects, like dry mouth or drowsiness, which are normal. Do you have any concerns or questions before we begin?"

3. Perform Hand Hygiene and Assess the Application Site

- Wash hands thoroughly and assess the patient's skin for an appropriate application site. Look for clean, dry, intact skin without redness, irritation, or hair.

What to say(while assessing):

- "I'll check your skin now to find a suitable area for the patch. It's important to avoid any areas with cuts, irritation, or excessive hair to ensure the medication absorbs properly."

4. Apply the Patch

- Follow manufacturer instructions to prepare and apply the patch. Peel the backing without touching the adhesive side, and firmly press it onto the selected area for the recommended time to ensure adherence.

What to say:

- "I'm applying the patch now. It needs to be placed securely on your skin, so it stays in place and works effectively. I'll ensure it's properly adhered to and that you're comfortable."

5. Educate the Patient

- Explain how to care for the patch, such as avoiding excessive water exposure, not touching or tampering with it, and monitoring for side effects. Provide instructions on when and how to replace the patch if required.

What to say:

↳ "Please avoid scratching or touching the patch. You can shower as usual but try not to submerge it in water for too long. If you notice redness, swelling, or any discomfort near the patch, let us know immediately. This patch needs to be replaced every three days, and we'll handle the replacements for you."

6. Monitor and Document

↳ Document the date, time, site of application, and patient education in the medical records. Monitor the patient for any adverse reactions.

What to say:

↳ "I've applied the patch and will record it in your chart now. I'll check on you regularly to ensure it's working as intended and that you're not experiencing any issues. If you feel any discomfort, please let me know."

연습 Scenario 2:
Inhalation Medication Administration

* Time: 10 minutes
* Setting: Outpatient Clinic
* Situation: A patient requires a dose of bronchodilator (Salbutamol) via a Spacer for asthma management, necessitating proper technique and education.

Example Scenario Description:

You are a nurse in an outpatient clinic. Mr. Daniel Smith, a 45-year-old patient with a history of asthma, is experiencing shortness of breath and wheezing. The doctor has prescribed Salbutamol, a bronchodilator, to be administered via a spacer. This scenario evaluates your ability to administer inhalation medication, educate the patient on proper technique, and monitor for adverse reactions.

Candidate Instructions:

1. Verify the Medication Order and Check Patient Identity

⤳ Confirm the prescription for Salbutamol and ensure the correct dose. Verify the patient's identity using two identifiers, such as name and date of birth.

What to say:

⤳ "Good morning, Mr. Smith. My name is [Your Name], and I'll assist you with your asthma medication today. To confirm, could you please tell me your full name and date of birth? Thank you. I'll be administering a bronchodilator, Salbutamol, which will help open your airways and make it easier for you to breathe."

2. Explain the Procedure and Obtain Consent

⤳ Describe how the Spacer works, its benefits, and any possible side effects. Obtain the patient's verbal consent to proceed.

What to say:

⤳ "This inhaler contains medication that will quickly relieve your asthma symptoms. You might feel a slight nervous or a faster heartbeat after using it, which is normal. Let me show you how to use it properly. Do you have any concerns or questions before we start?"

3. Perform Hand Hygiene and Prepare the Medication

⤳ Wash hands thoroughly to maintain hygiene. Shake the metered dose inhaler(MDI) well to ensure the medication is properly mixed.

What to say(while shaking the inhaler):

⤳ "I'm preparing the inhaler now by shaking it. This helps mix the medication evenly for effective delivery."

4. Assist the Patient in Using the Spacer

⤳ Instruct and assist the patient in using the inhaler correctly:
- Remove the cap from the inhaler and ensure it is clean
- Attach the inhaler to the spacer securely
- Ask the patient to exhale fully to empty their lungs
- Position the spacer between their lips, ensuring a tight seal
- Press the inhaler to release the medication into the spacer
- Instruct the patient to inhale slowly and deeply through the mouthpiece
- Ask the patient to hold their breath for approximately 10 seconds to allow the medication to reach the lungs, then instruct them to exhale slowly

What to say:

↳ "Let's take it step by step. First, take a deep breath out to empty your lungs. Now, place the spacer mouthpiece between your lips and make sure you're sealing it tightly. When I press the inhaler, inhale slowly and deeply through your mouth. Good. now hold your breath for about 10 seconds to let the medication work. Great! Now you can exhale slowly. Well done!"

5. Document and Educate

↳ Record the medication, dose, time, and any observations in the patient's medical record. Provide education on proper inhaler use, care, and when to seek help.

What to say:

↳ "I've recorded the administration in your chart. It's important to shake the inhaler each time before use and to rinse your mouth afterwards to prevent irritation. If your symptoms worsen or you feel this medication isn't working, please seek medical attention immediately. Do you have any questions about using your inhaler?"

6. Monitor for Adverse Reactions

↳ Observe the patient for any side effects, such as tremors or increased heart rate, and reassure them as needed.

What to say:

↳ "I'll stay with you for a few minutes to make sure you're feeling better and not experiencing any side effects. If you feel anything unusual, let me know right away."

연습 Scenario 3:
Clexane Injection after Total Hip Replacement (THR) due to Clotting Factor Disorder

* Time: 10 minutes
* Setting: Surgical Ward
* Situation: Clexane (Enoxaparin) Injection Post-Total Hip Replacement (THR)

Example Scenario Description:

You are a registered nurse working in the surgical ward. Your patient, Mr. George Smith, a 68-year-old male, has recently undergone a total hip replacement (THR) surgery. Mr. Smith has a clotting factor disorder, and the doctor has prescribed Clexane (Enoxaparin) injections as part of his post-operative care to prevent venous thromboembolism (VTE). Your task is to administer the Clexane injection, ensuring correct technique and patient safety.

Candidate Instructions:

1. Introduce yourself, Verify Medication Order and Check Patient Identity

- Knock on the door, greet the patient.
- Cross-check the doctor's prescription and the medication provided. Follow the "7 Rights of Medication Administration" (Right Patient, Right Drug, Right Dose, Right Route, Right Purpose, Right Time, Right documentation). Use two identifiers (e.g., name and date of birth) to confirm patient identity.

What to say:

- "Good morning, Mr. Smith. My name is [Your Name], and I'm your nurse today. Can I confirm your name and date of birth? Thank you."

2. Explain the Medication and Procedure

- Explain the purpose of the Clexane injection, how it helps prevent blood clots, and the procedure you will follow to administer it.

What to say:

- "I'll be administering an injection of Clexane (Enoxaparin) today. This is a blood thinner that will help prevent blood clots after your hip replacement surgery. It's important that we give it to you every day as prescribed. The injection will be given into the fatty tissue just under your skin, usually in your abdomen or thigh. You may feel a little sting when I inject the medication, but it should not be painful. Do you have any questions or concerns?"

: Obtain verbal consent before proceeding.

3. Ensure Patient Comfort and Positioning

↝ Ensure the patient is comfortable and positioned in a way that allows easy access to the injection site. Typically, the injection will be given in the abdomen, 2 inches away from the umbilicus, or in the thigh.

What to say:

↝ "Please lie back or sit in a comfortable position, and I'll prepare the injection now."

4. Perform Hand Hygiene and Wear PPE

↝ Wash your hands thoroughly and wear gloves to prevent contamination during the procedure.

What to say:

↝ "I'm now washing my hands and putting on gloves to ensure everything is sterile for your injection."

5. Prepare the Injection Site

↝ Clean the chosen injection site (usually the lower abdomen or thigh) with an alcohol swab to reduce the risk of infection.

What to say:

↝ "I'm cleaning the injection site with an alcohol swab to ensure it is sterile."

6. Administer the Clexane Injection

- Remove the protective cap from the syringe. Pinch the skin around the injection site to create a fold, and insert the needle at a 90-degree angle into the fatty tissue. Inject the medication slowly and steadily. Do not aspirate (pull back on the plunger) once the needle is inserted.
- After the injection, remove the needle quickly and apply gentle pressure to the site with a gauze pad. Do not rub the area.

What to say:

- "Now I'm going to insert the needle and give you the injection. It may feel a bit cold, but try to relax. I'll inject it slowly."

7. Dispose of Needle and Syringe Safely

- Immediately dispose of the needle and syringe in a sharp's container.

What to say:

- "I'm now disposing of the needle and syringe in the sharps container to ensure your safety."

8. Post-Procedure Care and Monitoring

8.1 Monitor for Immediate Reactions

- Observe the patient for any signs of immediate reactions to the injection, such as dizziness, nausea, or allergic responses. Ensure the injection site is not bleeding excessively.

What to say:

↳ "How are you feeling, Mr. Smith? You may notice a small bruise at the injection site, but it shouldn't cause significant discomfort. Please let me know if you experience any unusual reactions."

8.2 Assess the Injection Site

↳ Check the injection site for any signs of redness, swelling, or bleeding. If there is significant bruising or swelling, it may indicate an adverse reaction.

What to say:

↳ "I'll check the injection site to make sure there's no excessive bleeding or irritation."

9. Patient Education and Follow-Up Care

9.1 Educate the Patient on Clexane and Safety

↳ Educate the patient about the purpose of the medication, the importance of daily injections, and potential side effects such as bruising or irritation at the injection site.

What to say:

↳ "Clexane helps prevent blood clots, which is especially important after surgery. You may experience some bruising at the injection site, but this is normal. If you notice any unusual symptoms, such as excessive bruising, dizziness, or a rash, contact the nursing team immediately."

9.2 Advise on Injection Technique(if applicable)

↪ If the patient will be administering their own injections at home, provide instructions on how to give the injection safely, emphasizing the importance of rotating injection sites to avoid irritation.

What to say:

↪ "If you're going to be giving yourself injections at home, make sure to rotate the injection sites between your abdomen and thighs. It's important not to inject in the same spot each time to avoid irritation."

9.3 Schedule Follow-Up and Monitoring

↪ Remind the patient about any follow-up appointments or tests, including monitoring for signs of bleeding or bruising, and the need for regular blood tests to monitor the effects of the medication.

What to say:

↪ "Please come back for your next check-up as scheduled. We will also monitor your progress and make sure the Clexane is working effectively. Let us know if you have any concerns before your next visit."

10. Documentation and Reporting

↳ Record the time and date of the Clexane injection, the site of administration, and any observations or complications.

Example Documentation:

↳ "Administered 40mg Clexane(Enoxaparin) subcutaneously to Mr. George Smith in the lower abdomen at 10:00 AM. No complications noted, patient tolerated the procedure well."

# 연습 Scenario 4:
Insulin Doses Calculation and Administration(Long-Acting vs. Short-Acting Insulin)

* Time: 10 minutes
* Setting: Medical Ward
* Situation: Insulin Dose Calculation and Administration

✍ Example Scenario Description:

You are a registered nurse working in a medical ward. Your patient, Mrs. Evelyn Jones, a 72-year-old female with type 2 diabetes, requires insulin administration to control her blood glucose levels. You need to calculate the appropriate insulin doses based on her current blood glucose level and determine whether long-acting or short-acting insulin is required. Your task is to correctly calculate the insulin doses, choose the appropriate type (long-acting vs. short-acting), and administer the medication using the correct technique.

Candidate Instructions:

Step 1: Patient Communication and Preparation

1.1 Introduce Yourself and Confirm Identity

↣ Knock on the door, greet the patient, and confirm their identity using two identifiers (e.g., full name and date of birth).

What to say:

↣ "Good morning, Mrs. Jones. My name is [Your Name], and I am your nurse today. Could you please confirm your full name and date of birth? Thank you."

1.2 Explain the Medication and Procedure

↣ Explain the insulin therapy and the purpose of insulin injections in managing her diabetes. Discuss the difference between long-acting and short-acting insulin.

What to say:

↣ "I'm going to administer your insulin injection now. Insulin helps your body manage blood glucose levels. Long-acting insulin provides a steady level throughout the day, while short-acting insulin helps control blood glucose levels after meals. Based on your current blood glucose reading, I'll determine the appropriate type and dose of insulin."

: Obtain verbal consent before proceeding.

1.3 Ensure Patient Comfort and Positioning
- Ensure the patient is comfortably positioned, typically sitting or lying down, with easy access to the injection site (usually the abdomen or thigh).

What to say:
- "Please sit comfortably or lie back while I prepare the insulin injection."

Step 2: Perform Hand Hygiene and Wear PPE
- Wash your hands thoroughly and wear gloves to prevent contamination during the procedure.

What to say:
- "I'm now washing my hands and putting on gloves to ensure everything is sterile for your injection."

Step 3: Insulin Dose Calculation

3.1 Review Blood Glucose Level
- Obtain the patient's most recent blood glucose level (e.g., from a glucometer or lab results). Let's assume the patient's blood glucose is 14 mmol/L.

3.2 Calculate Insulin Dose
- Calculate the insulin dose based on the patient's blood glucose level and current insulin regimen. In New Zealand, correction insulin (additional doses of rapid-acting insulin) is used to manage pre-meal hyperglycaemia. The dose is calculated using the following formula:

- Correction Dose (units) = (Current Blood Glucose − Target Blood Glucose) ÷ Correction Factor
- The Correction Factor indicates how much 1 unit of insulin will lower the blood glucose level and is often estimated as 2.8 mmol/L for many patients. However, this can vary based on individual insulin sensitivity.
- Example Calculation:
    * Current Blood Glucose: 14 mmol/L
    * Target Blood Glucose: 8 mmol/L
    * Correction Factor: 2.8 mmol/L per unit of insulin
    * Correction Dose: (14 mmol/L − 8 mmol/L) ÷ 2.8 mmol/L per unit = 6 mmol/L ÷ 2.8 mmol/L per unit ≈ 2 units

What to say:

➢ "Your current blood glucose level is 14 mmol/L. To bring it down to our target of 8 mmol/L, I'll administer an additional 2 units of rapid-acting insulin."

3.3 Determine Insulin Type (Long-Acting or Short-Acting)

➢ Based on the patient's blood glucose level and doctor's orders, determine which type of insulin is appropriate. For the given scenario, the patient needs short-acting (rapid-acting) insulin to correct the elevated blood glucose level before meals.

What to say:
- "Since your blood glucose level is elevated before your meal, I'll administer rapid-acting insulin to quickly lower your blood glucose."

Step 4: Insulin Administration

4.1 Prepare the Injection Site
- Clean the injection site (usually the abdomen or thigh) with an alcohol swab to reduce the risk of infection.

What to say:
- "I'm cleaning the injection site with an alcohol swab to ensure it is sterile."

4.2 Prepare the Insulin Syringe or Pen
- If using a syringe, draw up the correct dose of rapid-acting insulin from the vial. If using an insulin pen, attach the needle and dial the correct dose.

What to say:
- "I'm now preparing the insulin for your injection. Please let me know if you feel uncomfortable."

4.3 Administer the Insulin Injection
- Pinch the skin of the injection site to create a fold. Insert the needle at a 90-degree angle into the fatty tissue, and slowly inject the insulin. Once the injection is complete, remove the needle and apply gentle pressure to the site with a gauze pad.

What to say:

↳ "I'm inserting the needle now and administering the insulin. It should be quick and relatively painless."

4.4 Dispose of the Needle and Syringe Safely

↳ Immediately dispose of the used syringe or pen needle in a sharps container.

What to say:

↳ "I'm now disposing of the needle in the sharps container for safety."

Step 5: Post-Procedure Care and Monitoring

5.1 Monitor for Immediate Reactions

↳ Observe the patient for any immediate reactions such as dizziness, shortness of breath, or swelling. These can be signs of hypoglycaemia (low blood glucose) or an allergic reaction.

What to say:

↳ "How are you feeling now? You should start feeling better shortly, but let me know if you experience any unusual symptoms."

5.2 Assess the Injection Site

↳ Check the injection site for any redness, swelling, or signs of infection.

What to say:

↳ "I'll check the injection site to ensure there is no irritation or excessive swelling."

Step 6: Patient Education and Follow-Up Care

6.1 Educate the Patient on Insulin Management

➣ Educate the patient about insulin therapy, including the importance of taking insulin regularly, monitoring blood glucose levels, and recognizing signs of hypoglycemia.

What to say:

➣ "It's important to take your insulin at the same time every day. You should also monitor your blood sugar levels regularly to ensure the insulin is working. If you notice any symptoms of low blood sugar, such as shakiness or dizziness, let us know immediately."

6.2 Advise on Diet and Lifestyle

➣ Advise the patient about the importance of maintaining a healthy diet and exercise regimen in conjunction with insulin therapy.

What to say:

➣ "Be mindful of your diet and try to maintain a balanced meal plan. Exercise can also help with managing your blood sugar levels."

6.3 Schedule Follow-Up and Monitoring

➣ Remind the patient about any follow-up appointments or lab tests for blood glucose levels.

What to say:

➣ "Please come back for your next follow-up visit so we can check how well your insulin is working. We'll also monitor your blood sugar levels and make adjustments if needed."

Step 7: Documentation and Reporting

7.1 Document the Medication Administration

↳ Record the time and date of the insulin administration, the dose, type of insulin, and the injection site. Document the patient's blood glucose level and any observations or complications.

Example Documentation:

↳ "Administered 7 units of short-acting insulin subcutaneously to Mrs. Evelyn Jones at 10:30 AM. Blood glucose level before administration was 250 mg/dL. No complications noted, patient tolerated the procedure well."

7.2 Report Any Adverse Reactions

↳ If the patient experiences side effects such as hypoglycemia or allergic reactions, report these to the doctor immediately.

What to say:

↳ "I've documented the insulin administration and will report any unusual findings or reactions to the medical team for further evaluation."

❽ 의사소통 및 팀워크

Station Eight: Communication and teamwork

* **Time:** 10 minutes
* **Setting:** Inpatient Ward
* **Situation:** You are ending your shift and need to hand over the care of your patients to the incoming nurse.

✐ Example Example Scenario Description:

You are a registered nurse finishing your shift on an inpatient ward. You are responsible for handing over the care of your assigned patients to the incoming nurse. This task involves using the ISBAR(Identity, Situation, Background, Assessment, Recommendation) format to ensure that critical information is clearly communicated, enabling a smooth transition of care. This scenario evaluates your ability to provide an effective handover and ensure continuity of care.

당신은 병동에서 근무하는 간호사로써 근무를 마칠때, 자신에게 배정되었던 환자들의 케어를 다음 교대 근무 간호사에게 인계해야 합니다. ISBAR(Identity, Situation, Background, Assessment, Recommendation) 형식을 사용하여 중요한 정보를 명확하게 전달하고, 원활한 치료 전환을 보장해야 합니다. 이 시나리오는 효과적인 인계 과정을 제공하고 치료의 연속성을 보장하는 능력을 평가합니다.

Candidate Instructions:

1. Prepare a Structured Handover Using SBAR Format

Tasks:

- Organize the information for each patient into the ISBAR format:
    - **Identity:** your name, role, department(if they don't know you), Patient's name, age and location
    - **Situation:** Patient's diagnosis, and current issue.
    - **Background**: Relevant medical history and treatment received during your shift.
    - **Assessment:** Current condition, including vital signs, pain levels, physical assessment result, and any recent changes.
    - **Recommendation:** Next steps in care, such as pending tests, follow-up treatments, or potential concerns.

What to Say:

- "Let's start with Patient A. They are a 65-year-old male admitted for pneumonia. During my shift, their oxygen saturation dropped to 88%, requiring an increase in supplemental oxygen. Their vital signs

are now stable, but their respiratory rate is still slightly elevated."
- "I recommend monitoring their oxygen levels closely and administering the prescribed nebulizer treatment in the next hour."

> 먼저 환자 A부터 시작하겠습니다. 환자 A는 65세 남성으로 폐렴으로 입원하셨습니다. 제 근무 시간 동안 환자의 산소 포화도가 88%로 떨어져서 보조 산소를 증가시켜야 했습니다. 현재 vital sign은 안정적이나, 호흡수가 여전히 약간 상승해 있습니다. 환자의 산소 수준을 면밀히 모니터링하고, 다음 한 시간 내에 처방된 네뷸라이저 치료를 시행해야 될것으로 보입니다."

2. Clearly and Concisely Communicate Each Patient's Status

Tasks:
- Provide a brief summary of each patient, including their current status, ongoing treatments, and any notable changes during your shift.
- Use precise language to ensure the incoming nurse understands the key points.

> 각 환자에 대한 간략한 요약을 제공하며, 현재 상태, 진행 중인 치료 및 근무 시간 동안의 중요한 변화를 포함합니다.
> 정확한 언어를 사용하여 인계를 받는 간호사가 주요 사항을 잘 이해할 수 있도록 합니다.

What to Say:
- "Patient B is a 72-year-old female recovering from hip surgery. She has been mobilized with assistance today and reports moderate pain at the incision site,

which is managed with analgesics. There's no sign of infection at the wound site."
- "Please ensure she continues to receive her pain medication as scheduled and assist her with mobilization as tolerated."

> 환자 B는 고관절 수술 후 회복 중인 72세 여성입니다. 오늘 도움을 받아 보행했으며, 절개 부위에 중등도의 통증을 호소했으나 진통제로 관리되고 있습니다. 상처 부위에 감염 징후는 없습니다."
> "진통제를 예정대로 계속 투여하고, 환자가 가능한 한 보행을 할수있도록 도와주세요."

3. Ensure the Incoming Nurse Understands Critical Information

Tasks:
- Allow time for the incoming nurse to ask questions and clarify any details.
- Confirm that they are aware of any urgent or time-sensitive tasks.

> 인계를 받는 간호사가 질문을 하고 세부 사항을 명확히 할 수 있는 시간을 제공하세요. 그 간호사가 긴급하거나 시간에 민감한 일에 대해 알고 있는지 확인하세요.

What to Say:
- "Do you have any questions about Patient C's medication changes? It's important that their anticoagulant is given on time due to their recent DVT."

> "If anything is unclear or if you need further information later, feel free to contact me before I leave."

> "Patient C의 약물 변경 사항에 대해 질문이 있나요? 최근 발생한 deep vein thrombosis(DVT) 때문에 항응고제가 정시간에 투여되는 것이 중요합니다."
> "혹시 불명확한 점이 있거나 추가 정보가 필요하면 제가 퇴근하기 전에 언제든지 연락하세요."

4. Document the Handover Accurately

Tasks:

↳ Record the details of the handover in the appropriate format or system, ensuring it is clear and complete.

↳ Include any significant updates, changes in treatment, and recommendations for the next shift.

> "적절한 형식이나 시스템에 따라 인수인계 세부사항을 기록하고, 명확하고 완전하게 작성합니다."
> "주요 업데이트, 치료 변경 사항, 그리고 다음 교대를 위한 권고사항을 포함합니다."

*What to Say:

↳ "I've documented all patient updates in the handover sheet. You'll find specific details about pending tasks and test results there as well."

↳ "Please review the documentation before starting your assessments to ensure nothing is missed."

> "환자 업데이트 내용을 모두 인수인계 기록지에 작성했습니다. 대기 중인 업무와 검사 결과에 대한 세부 사항도 거기에 있습니다."
> "환자 사정을 시작하기 전에 제 노트를 검토하여 누락된 사항이 없는지 확인해주세요."

연습 Scenario 1:
Patient Education

* Time: 15 minutes
* Setting: Outpatient Clinic ? Consultation Room
* Situation: A patient has been newly diagnosed with type 2 diabetes and requires comprehensive education on managing their condition at home.

Example Scenario Description:

You are a registered nurse in an outpatient clinic. Mr. Steven Walker, a 52-year-old male, has been diagnosed with type 2 diabetes after presenting with fatigue, increased thirst, and frequent urination. His fasting blood glucose was 160 mg/dL, and his HbA1c is 8.2%. Mr. Walker has limited knowledge about diabetes management and is feeling overwhelmed about making lifestyle changes. This scenario evaluates your ability to educate and empower the patient to manage their condition effectively at home.

Candidate Instructions:

1. Explain the Basics of Diabetes Management

Tasks

- Educate the patient on the importance of blood glucose monitoring, a balanced diet, regular exercise, and taking prescribed medications.
- Use simple language and visuals(if available) to explain complex concepts like blood sugar levels and insulin resistance.

* What to Say:

- "Diabetes means your body has trouble managing the sugar in your blood. We'll focus on keeping your blood sugar levels within a healthy range to prevent complications."
- "Monitoring your blood sugar regularly is important because it helps you see how food, exercise, and medication affect your levels. You'll use a glucometer for this. I'll show you how it works."
- "A balanced diet is key. You'll want to include foods like whole grains, vegetables, lean proteins, and healthy fats while limiting sugary and processed foods. Small, regular meals can help keep your blood sugar stable."
- "Exercise is just as important. Even a 30-minute walk most days can make a big difference in lowering your blood sugar and improving your health."

2. Demonstrate Blood Glucose Monitoring and Medication Use

Tasks
- Provide a step-by-step demonstration of how to use a glucometer to check blood glucose levels.
- Explain the purpose of prescribed medications(e.g., metformin) and the importance of taking them as directed.

What to Say:
- "Let me show you how to use your glucometer. First, wash your hands, then insert a test strip into the meter. Use the lancet to prick your finger, place the blood drop on the strip, and wait for the reading. It's simple once you've practised a few times."
- "Your doctor has prescribed metformin to help your body use insulin more effectively. It's important to take it with meals to avoid an upset stomach. Let's set up a schedule that works for you."

3. Use Teach-Back to Ensure Understanding

Tasks
- Ask the patient to repeat key information to confirm they understand the concepts and skills you've explained.
- Clarify any misconceptions or confusion.

What to Say:

↪ "Can you walk me through how you'll check your blood sugar at home? What steps will you take?"

↪ "Can you explain why it's important to take your medication as prescribed and how you'll include exercise in your routine?"

↪ "Let's talk about your meals. What kind of foods do you think you can include more of to keep your blood sugar steady?"

4. Provide Written Materials and Resources

Tasks

↪ Hand out easy-to-read pamphlets or booklets on diabetes management, meal planning, and exercise tips.

↪ Offer information about local diabetes education programs or support groups.

What to Say:

↪ "Here's a booklet that explains everything we talked about today, including meal ideas and tips for staying active. It also has a chart where you can log your blood sugar readings."

↪ "If you'd like, I can connect you with a diabetes educator or a support group in our area. They can provide additional guidance and encouragement."

5. Encourage Questions and Provide Empathetic Responses

Tasks
- Create a safe and welcoming environment for the patient to ask questions.
- Address concerns with clear and empathetic explanations.

What to Say:
- "I know this can feel like a lot to take in, but you're not alone in this. Do you have any questions about anything we've discussed so far?"
- "It's completely normal to feel overwhelmed at first. We'll take it step by step, and I'm here to support you every step of the way."
- "If you're worried about any specific part of this, like using the glucometer or making diet changes, let's talk about it and figure out a solution together."

연습 Scenario 2:
Conflict Resolution

* Time: 10 minutes
* Setting: Nursing Station ? Inpatient Unit
* Situation: A disagreement arises between two team members regarding the best approach to managing a patient's care. As the nurse responsible for facilitating teamwork, you need to address the conflict professionally, ensuring patient care remains the priority.

Example Scenario Description:

You are a registered nurse in an inpatient unit. During a team discussion, two colleagues, a nurse and a physiotherapist, have differing opinions on the approach to Mr. John Adams' care. Mr. Adams, a 72-year-old recovering from a stroke, requires both effective mobility support and careful management of his blood pressure. The nurse prioritizes frequent monitoring and rest, while the physiotherapist emphasizes the importance of early mobilization. This scenario evaluates your ability to mediate conflict, ensure a collaborative approach, and maintain focus on high-quality patient care.

Candidate Instructions:

1. Facilitate a Calm and Respectful Discussion

Tasks

- Acknowledge the disagreement and create a safe environment for open communication.
- Set ground rules for a respectful and professional discussion.

What to Say:

- "I understand there's a difference in opinions about Mr. Adams' care. Let's take a moment to discuss this calmly and focus on what's best for the patient."
- "I'd like us to approach this with mutual respect. Each of you will have the chance to share your perspective, and we'll work together to find the best solution."

2. Encourage Each Person to Express Their Views

Tasks

- Allow each team member to explain their reasoning and concerns without interruption.
- Actively listen and validate their perspectives.

What to Say:

➢ To the nurse: "Can you explain why you feel frequent monitoring and rest are most important for Mr. Adams right now?"

➢ To the physiotherapist: "Can you share your perspective on the benefits of early mobilization in his recovery?"

➢ "Thank you both for sharing your insights. It's clear that both approaches have valid points that could benefit Mr. Adams."

3. Help the Team Find Common Ground

Tasks

➢ Highlight shared goals, such as optimizing the patient's recovery and minimizing risks.

➢ Facilitate brainstorming to develop a care plan that incorporates elements of both perspectives.

What to Say:

➢ "Both of you are advocating for Mr. Adams' recovery, which is our common goal. Let's explore how we can balance careful monitoring with early mobilization."

➢ "What if we schedule short, guided mobility sessions at times when his vital signs are stable? This way, we can address both safety and physical recovery."

4. Reflect on the Importance of Communication and Teamwork

Tasks

- Summarize the agreed-upon plan and emphasize how collaboration ensures high-quality care.
- Discuss how resolving conflicts constructively improves team dynamics and patient outcomes.

What to Say:

- "Thank you both for sharing your expertise and working together to create a plan for Mr. Adams. Your collaboration ensures he receives the best possible care."
- "Effective communication and teamwork are essential in healthcare. By combining our strengths and expertise, we can achieve the best outcomes for our patients."

연습 Scenario 3:
Crisis Communication

* Time: 10 minutes
* Setting: Medical Ward
* Situation: A patient under your care suddenly deteriorates, requiring urgent intervention. You must act quickly to escalate care, provide immediate support, and ensure effective communication with the healthcare team.

Example Scenario Description:

You are a registered nurse working on a busy medical ward. Mr. Thomas Brown, a 67-year-old patient admitted for pneumonia, suddenly becomes acutely unwell. His oxygen saturation has dropped to 85%, he is experiencing shortness of breath, and his respiratory rate has increased to 30 breaths per minute. His skin appears pale and clammy. This scenario evaluates your ability to respond promptly and appropriately in a medical emergency by following emergency protocols, effectively communicating, and ensuring optimal teamwork.

Candidate Instructions:

1. Recognize and Communicate the Emergency

Task
- Assess the situation and recognize the signs of acute respiratory distress.
- Activate the emergency protocol by calling for the rapid response team(RRT) or code team.
- Clearly and concisely communicate the patient's condition using an established framework(e.g., ISBAR: Identity, Situation, Background, Assessment, Recommendation).

What to Say:
- "I'm calling for urgent help. This is Mr. Thomas Brown, a 67-year-old male with pneumonia. His oxygen saturation has dropped to 85%, respiratory rate is 30, and he appears pale and clammy. I'm concerned about respiratory failure. Please respond immediately."

2. Provide Immediate Care and Delegate Tasks

Tasks
- Initiate immediate interventions to stabilize the patient(e.g., elevate the head of the bed, administer supplemental oxygen).

- Delegate tasks to available team members(e.g., assigning someone to monitor vital signs, prepare emergency equipment, or notify the physician).

What to Say:
- "Can you please elevate the head of the bed to improve his breathing? I'll start administering oxygen."
- "I need someone to stay with the patient and monitor his vital signs while I prepare to report to the physician."
- "Can you please grab the emergency equipment and check his recent blood gas results?"

3. Participate in a Team Response

Tasks
- Support the rapid response team or other healthcare providers upon their arrival.
- Provide a clear handover, updating the team on any interventions you initiated and recent changes in the patient's condition.

What to Say:
- "Before you arrived, we elevated the head of the bed and started oxygen at 8 L/min. His saturation has improved slightly to 88%, but his respiratory rate remains high at 30 breaths per minute."

➼ "He was stable during the previous hour, with oxygen saturation at 94% on 4 L/min. This deterioration was sudden."

4. Participate in a Debriefing Session

Tasks

➼ Join the team after the crisis to discuss the event. Reflect on what went well, what challenges arose, and how the response could improve.
➼ Identify areas for improvement, including communication, preparedness, or response times.

What to Say:

➼ "It was helpful that we escalated care quickly and initiated oxygen therapy early. However, we could have had the emergency equipment closer to the bedside for faster access."
➼ "I think the communication between team members was clear, but we could review ways to ensure the rapid response team is notified even faster during busy shifts."

연습 Scenario 4:
Communicating with a Patient with Limited English Proficiency

* **Time**: 10 minutes
* **Setting**: General Ward
* **Situation**: A patient with limited English proficiency is admitted, and you must ensure effective communication to provide safe and patient-centred care.

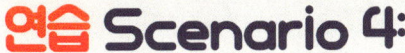 Example Scenario Description:

You are a registered nurse caring for Mrs. Maria Hernandez, a 55-year-old female recently admitted with symptoms of dehydration and confusion. She is fluent in Spanish but speaks limited English, and her family is unavailable to translate at the moment. This scenario evaluates your ability to communicate effectively using appropriate tools and strategies to ensure she understands her care plan and feels supported.

Candidate Instructions:

1. Establish Effective Communication

Tasks

- Use translation services(e.g., phone or video interpreter services) to communicate with the patient.
- Speak slowly, use simple language, and avoid medical jargon.
- Observe nonverbal cues, such as facial expressions and body language, to gauge understanding.

What to Say:

- "Good morning, Mrs. Hernandez. I'm your nurse today. I want to make sure we understand each other, so I'll connect us with an interpreter to help us communicate clearly."
- To the interpreter: "Please ask Mrs. Hernandez how she is feeling today and if she has any pain."

2. Provide Patient Education and Confirm Understanding

Tasks

- Explain her condition and treatment plan using the interpreter, ensuring she understands what is happening and what care she will receive.
- Use the teach-back method to confirm understanding by asking her to repeat key points in her own words(via the interpreter).

What to Say:

↬ "Mrs. Hernandez, you are here because you were dehydrated. We'll give you fluids through an IV to help you feel better."

↬ "Can you explain back to me, in your own words, why we are giving you the IV fluids? I want to make sure everything is clear."

3. Respect Cultural Preferences and Address Concerns

Tasks

↬ Ask if there are any cultural or personal preferences regarding her care.

↬ Listen actively and empathetically to her concerns, using the interpreter to provide reassurance and solutions.

What to Say:

↬ "Mrs. Hernandez, is there anything about your care that we should know to make you more comfortable? For example, any preferences about meals, medications, or how we can support you?"

↬ "It's very important to me that you feel safe and comfortable. Please let us know if you have any concerns or questions."

4. Document and Collaborate with the Team

Tasks

↣ Document the use of the interpreter, key points discussed, and any preferences or concerns raised.

↣ Communicate with the healthcare team about the patient's language needs and preferences to ensure continuity of care.

What to Say to Team Members:

↣ "Mrs. Hernandez is more comfortable communicating in Spanish. I used the phone interpreter service to explain her condition and care plan. She understands and has no additional concerns at this time."

↣ "Please ensure the interpreter service is used for any future discussions or education until her family is available."

⑨ 간호계획 수립

Station nine: Planning nursing care

* Time: 10 minutes
* Setting: General Surgical ward
* Situation: A patient has just undergone abdominal surgery and requires comprehensive postoperative care.

✏ Example Example Scenario Description:

You are a registered nurse in a General surgical ward. Mrs. Sarah Thompson, a 58-year-old female patient, has just undergone an abdominal surgery(e.g., colectomy). You are tasked with assessing her condition, developing a postoperative care plan, and ensuring she and her family are well-informed and supported in the recovery process. This scenario evaluates your ability to assess a patient's postoperative condition and create a comprehensive care plan to ensure proper recovery.

당신은 일반외과 병동 간호사입니다. 58세 여성 환자인 사라 톰슨(Mrs. Sarah Thompson)은 복부 수술(예: 결장 절제술)을 방금 마친 상태입니다. 당신은 그녀의 상태를 평가하고, 수술 후 간호 계획을 수립하며, 그녀와 그녀의 가족이 회복 과정에서 충분한 정보를 제공받고 지원을 받을 수 있도록 해야 합니다. 이 시나리오는 환자의 수술 후 상태를 평가하고 적절한 회복을 보장하기 위한 포괄적인 간호 계획을 수립할 수 있는 능력을 평가합니다.

Candidate Instructions:

1. Conduct a Thorough Assessment of the Postoperative Condition

- Assess vital signs(blood pressure, heart rate, respiratory rate, temperature) and pain level.
- Examine the surgical incision for signs of infection(e.g., redness, swelling, drainage).
- Evaluate the patient's comfort and mobility level, noting any difficulty with movement or breathing.

활력 징후(혈압, 심박수, 호흡수, 체온)와 통증 수준을 평가하세요.
수술 절개 부위를 검사하여 감염 징후(예: 발적, 부기, 배액)가 있는지 확인하세요.
환자의 편안함과 보행 수준을 평가하며, 움직임이나 호흡에 어려움이 있는지 확인하세요.

What to say:

- "Good morning, Mrs. Thompson. I'm here to check on you after your surgery. I'll start by taking your vital signs to ensure you're recovering well."
- "I'll also examine your incision site to make sure there are no signs of infection. Are you feeling any pain or discomfort right now?"

> "안녕하세요, 톰슨 씨. 수술 후 몸상태가 어떠신지 확인하려합니다. 먼저 활력 징후를 측정하여 회복 상태가 좋은지 확인하겠습니다."
> "절개 부위에 감염 징후가 없는지 확인하려 하는데요, 현재 통증이나 불편함이 있으신가요?"

2. Develop a Care Plan

⤳ Plan for effective pain management, considering both pharmacological(e.g., analgesics) and non-pharmacological methods(e.g., positioning, relaxation).

⤳ Identify potential complications such as infection or deep vein thrombosis(DVT) and plan for early intervention.

⤳ Plan for early ambulation to promote circulation and prevent complications like pneumonia and DVT.

> 약물 치료(예: 진통제)와 비약물 치료(예: 자세 조정, 이완 요법)를 포함한 효과적인 통증 관리를 계획합니다.
> 감염이나 Deep Vein Thrombosis(DVT)과 같은 잠재적 합병증을 인지하고 조기 중재를 계획합니다.
> 순환을 촉진하고 폐렴 및 DVT와 같은 합병증을 예방하기 위해 조기 보행을 계획합니다.

What to say:

⤳ "We'll work together to manage your pain and make sure you're as comfortable as possible. I'll be administering medication to help manage any discomfort, and we'll also use positioning to minimize pain."

➤ "It's also important for you to start moving around as soon as we can to avoid potential complications. I'll assist you with gentle ambulation to help you regain strength and improve circulation."

"통증을 관리하고 환자분이 가능한 한 편안하게 지낼 수 있도록 저희 의료진은 함께 노력할 것입니다. 불편함을 줄이기 위해 약물을 투여할 것이며, 통증을 최소화하기 위해 자세를 조정하는 부분도 고려할 것입니다."
"잠재적 합병증을 예방하기 위해 가능한 빨리 움직이기 시작하는 것도 중요합니다. 제가 에너지와 혈액 순환을 개선할 수 있도록 보행을 도와 드리겠습니다."

3. Plan for Nutritional Support and Fluid Balance

➤ Plan for the initiation of a postoperative diet, starting with clear liquids and advancing to solid foods as tolerated.

➤ Ensure adequate fluid intake to prevent dehydration and promote wound healing.

"수술 후 식이 계획을 시작합니다. 먼저 맑은 액체부터 시작하고, 환자분께서 잘 소화를 시키시면 점차 고형식으로 진행합니다."
"탈수를 예방하고 상처 치유를 촉진하기 위해 적절한 수분 섭취를 보장합니다."

What to say:

➤ "We'll start you on clear liquids today to make sure your stomach is ready for food after surgery. Once you're able to tolerate that, we can move on to solid foods."

➤ "It's important to stay hydrated to support your recovery, so I'll monitor your fluid intake throughout the day."

> "오늘은 맑은 액체로 식사를 시작하겠습니다. 이는 수술 후 위가 음식을 받을 준비가 되었는지 확인하기 위한 것입니다. 이를 잘 소화하시면 고형식으로 진행할 수 있습니다."
>
> "회복을 돕기 위해 수분 섭취를 유지하는 것이 중요합니다. 하루 동안 수분 섭취량을 모니터링하겠습니다."

4. Communicate the Care Plan to the Patient and Family

- Clearly explain the care plan to the patient, ensuring they understand the postoperative instructions and the importance of follow-up care.
- Discuss potential complications and how to recognize signs of infection, bleeding, or other concerns.
- Provide the family with an understanding of the care plan and how they can support the patient's recovery at home.

> 환자에게 간호 계획을 명확히 설명하고, 퇴원 후 지침과 추후 관리의 중요성을 이해하도록 돕습니다. 발생할 수 있는 합병증 및 감염, 출혈 또는 기타 문제의 징후를 인식하는 방법에 대해 논의합니다. 가족에게 간호 계획에 대해 설명하고, 가정에서 환자의 회복을 지원할 수 있는 방법을 안내합니다.

What to say to the patient:

- "You'll need to follow some important instructions after you leave the hospital. This includes caring for your incision site, managing pain, and knowing when to seek medical help."
- "If you notice any changes, such as increased redness, swelling, or drainage from your incision, or

if you develop a fever, please let us know right away."

> "퇴원 후에는 몇 가지 중요한 지침을 따라야 합니다. 여기에는 절개 부위 관리, 통증 조절, 그리고 의료 도움이 필요할 때를 아는 것이 포함됩니다."
> "만약 절개 부위에 발적, 부기, 또는 분비물이 증가하거나, 발열이 발생하면 즉시 저희에게 알려주세요."

What to say to the family:

↪ "It's important that we work together to support Mrs. Thompson's recovery. She may need assistance with walking and managing her pain at home. I will provide you with specific instructions to ensure a smooth transition from hospital to home."

> 토마슨 씨의 회복을 돕기 위해 함께 노력하는 것이 중요합니다. 환자분은 집에서 보행부분과 통증 관리에 대한 지원이 필요할 수 있습니다. 병원에서 집으로 원활히 전환할 수 있도록 구체적인 지침을 제공해 드리겠습니다."

연습 Scenario 1:
Diabetes Management

* Time: 10 minutes
* Setting: Outpatient Clinic
* Situation: A newly diagnosed diabetic patient requires a comprehensive care plan to manage their condition.

✎ Example Scenario Description:

You are a registered nurse working in an outpatient clinic. Mr. David Nguyen, a 45-year-old male patient, has been recently diagnosed with type 2 diabetes. He is unsure about how to manage his condition and has limited knowledge regarding blood glucose monitoring, insulin administration, and dietary changes necessary to control his blood sugar levels. Your task is to assess his current understanding of diabetes, develop a comprehensive care plan to manage his condition and ensure that he has the tools and knowledge needed for self-management. This scenario evaluates your ability to educate the patient, develop an individualized care plan, and collaborate with other healthcare professionals to provide a holistic approach to diabetes management.

Candidate Instructions:

1. Assess the Patient's Knowledge About Diabetes and Management

- Ask the patient about their understanding of diabetes, including how it affects the body and the importance of blood glucose monitoring, insulin administration, and diet.
- Evaluate the patient's knowledge of the signs and symptoms of hyperglycaemia and hypoglycaemia.
- Identify any gaps in the patient's knowledge or misconceptions and address them in a compassionate and clear manner.

What to say:
- "Mr. Nguyen, can you tell me what you know about diabetes and how it affects your body?"
- "Do you understand how blood glucose monitoring works and why it's important to check your levels regularly?"
- "Have you been given any information about how insulin helps to regulate your blood sugar, and do you feel comfortable with administering it?"

2. Create a Comprehensive Care Plan for Diabetes Management

- Develop a care plan that includes patient education on how to properly monitor blood glucose levels, use insulin as prescribed, and make necessary dietary changes to maintain a healthy blood sugar level.
- Provide guidance on setting up a daily routine for monitoring blood glucose, taking insulin, and making appropriate food choices.
- Plan for setting realistic goals for blood glucose targets, activity levels, and weight management.

What to say:

- "To manage your diabetes effectively, you will need to monitor your blood sugar several times a day. I will show you how to use a blood glucose meter and explain how to interpret the readings."
- "You'll also need to follow a regular insulin schedule. I will demonstrate how to give yourself an injection and discuss when and how to adjust your doses."
- "A healthy diet is key to controlling your blood sugar. We will discuss the types of foods that are beneficial for you, and I'll help you make a plan for your meals."

3. Include Physical Activity as Part of the Care Plan

- Discuss the importance of regular physical activity in managing diabetes and how exercise helps to control blood glucose levels.

- Work with the patient to set achievable activity goals based on their current health status and preferences.
- Address any concerns or barriers the patient may have to incorporating physical activity into their daily routine.

What to say:
- "Regular exercise is essential for controlling your blood sugar and improving your overall health. What types of physical activities do you enjoy, or are you interested in trying?"
- "We will set a goal for you to engage in at least 30 minutes of moderate activity, like walking or swimming, most days of the week. It's important to start slow and gradually increase the intensity."
- "I understand that starting a new exercise routine can be challenging, but together we'll come up with a plan that fits into your lifestyle."

4. Collaborate with a Dietitian and Diabetes Educator

- Arrange for a consultation with a dietitian to provide additional guidance on meal planning and managing carbohydrate intake.
- Collaborate with a diabetes educator to offer further resources and education on how to live well with diabetes, including tips on managing blood sugar during illness or stress.

⤳ Provide the patient with written resources or direct them to local support groups to further assist with their self-management.

What to say:
⤳ "I've arranged for you to meet with our dietitian, who will help you develop a meal plan that supports your diabetes management."
⤳ "We also have a diabetes educator who can give you additional tips on how to manage your blood sugar and how to cope with any challenges you may face."
⤳ "I'll provide you with some written materials, and if you ever have questions, feel free to reach out. There are also support groups for people with diabetes where you can connect with others in similar situations."

연습 Scenario 2:
Palliative Care Plan

* Time: 10 minutes
* Setting: Palliative Care Unit
* Situation: A patient with advanced cancer is transitioning to palliative care.

✍ Example Scenario Description:

You are a registered nurse working in a palliative care unit. Mrs. Linda Davis, a 65-year-old patient with advanced stage cancer, has been referred to your unit for palliative care. She is experiencing significant physical discomfort, including pain, nausea, and anxiety, and has expressed concerns about the progression of her illness. Your task is to assess her physical, emotional, and spiritual needs holistically and develop a care plan that ensures her comfort and dignity during this stage of life. This scenario emphasizes the importance of providing compassionate, comprehensive care tailored to the patient's needs while collaborating with a multidisciplinary team.

Candidate Instructions:

1. Conduct a Holistic Assessment of the Patient's Needs

- Assess the patient's physical symptoms, including pain, nausea, and other discomforts related to her cancer diagnosis.
- Address the emotional impact of the diagnosis, such as anxiety, fear, or feelings of depression, and evaluate the need for psychological support.
- Consider the spiritual needs of the patient, including her values, beliefs, and any religious or cultural practices that may be important to her care.

What to say:

- "Mrs. Davis, I know this is a difficult time for you, and I want to make sure we address all aspects of your care. Can you describe the pain or discomfort you're feeling right now?"
- "I'd also like to know how you're feeling emotionally. Are there any concerns, fears, or thoughts you'd like to talk about?"
- "I understand that spiritual matters might be important to you at this time. Is there anything you'd like us to know or anyone you'd like to speak with for spiritual support?"

2. Develop a Care Plan Focused on Symptom Management

- Create a comprehensive care plan to manage the patient's symptoms, including strategies for pain control, nausea relief, and reducing anxiety.
- Implement pharmacological interventions such as opioids for pain relief, antiemetics for nausea, and anxiolytics for anxiety, ensuring to assess for any contraindications or interactions with current treatments.
- Address non-pharmacological interventions such as relaxation techniques, breathing exercises, and music therapy to enhance comfort.

What to say:

- "To help manage your pain, we will provide medications such as morphine or other opioids. This should help you feel more comfortable. Is there any particular time when you feel your pain is worse?"
- "We can also help manage your nausea with antiemetic medications. I'll make sure you have the right medications to help keep you comfortable."
- "In addition to medications, we can use techniques like deep breathing or listening to calming music. Would you like to try any of these methods to help with your anxiety?"

3. Coordinate Care with a Multidisciplinary Team

↝ Collaborate with palliative care specialists, social workers, and chaplains to ensure all aspects of the patient's care are addressed.
↝ Ensure that a plan for psychological support is in place to address any concerns regarding the end of life and to provide emotional comfort.
↝ Facilitate communication between healthcare providers to ensure that the patient's needs are met promptly and comprehensively.

What to say:

↝ "I'll coordinate with our palliative care specialists to make sure we have the best approach for managing your symptoms. We will also include a social worker who can help with any practical or emotional concerns you may have."
↝ "If you feel it would help, I can arrange for a chaplain to come and speak with you. They can offer spiritual support, regardless of your beliefs."
↝ "Together, we'll work to ensure your care is well-coordinated, so you can focus on being comfortable and surrounded by the support you need."

4. Communicate the Care Plan with the Patient and Their Family

- Discuss the goals of palliative care with the patient and her family, explaining that the focus is on comfort, dignity, and quality of life rather than curative treatment.
- Provide information on available support services, including social work, chaplain services, and hospice care if applicable.
- Address any questions or concerns the family may have about the transition to palliative care and ensure they understand the plan moving forward.

What to say:
- "Mrs. Davis, our goal is to ensure you're as comfortable as possible during this time, which means focusing on pain relief and emotional support, not necessarily curative treatments."
- "Your family will be an important part of this care, and I want to make sure they have all the information they need. We also have support services available, like counselling and chaplain services, that can help guide you all through this process."
- "If you have any questions or concerns, please don't hesitate to ask. Our team is here to support you, and we will make sure to adjust your care plan as your needs change."

연습 Scenario 3:
Paediatric Asthma Care Plan

* Time: 10 minutes
* Setting: Paediatric Outpatient Clinic
* Situation: A child with asthma is experiencing frequent exacerbations and needs a revised care plan.

Example Scenario Description:

You are a registered nurse working in a paediatric outpatient clinic. Alex, a 7-year-old child with asthma, has been experiencing frequent exacerbations despite being on standard asthma medication. The child's parents express concerns about the frequency and severity of these episodes and want to ensure better asthma management. Your task is to assess the child's current asthma management, develop a revised care plan to reduce exacerbations and provide the family with the education and resources they need to manage the condition effectively.

✍ Candidate Instructions:

1. Assess the Child's Current Asthma Management

- Begin by reviewing the child's asthma history, including frequency and severity of exacerbations, medication adherence, and use of inhalers.
- Assess for known triggers, such as allergens, smoke, or exercise, and ask the parents if they've identified any specific triggers.
- Discuss the effectiveness of the child's current medications(e.g., bronchodilators, corticosteroids) and whether they are being used as prescribed.

What to say:

- "Alex, can you tell me if you've had trouble breathing or coughing lately? How often does this happen?"
- "Let's talk about your asthma medications. Are you using your inhaler as prescribed, and have you noticed if it helps when you use it?"
- "I'd like to know about anything that might make your asthma worse, like pollen, dust, or even cold weather. Have you noticed any patterns in your symptoms?"

2. Develop a Revised Care Plan

- Based on the assessment, create a care plan that includes adjustments to the child's medication regimen. This might involve increasing the dosage of a rescue

inhaler, adding a long-term controller medication, or adjusting the type of inhaler.
- Address environmental modifications such as reducing exposure to allergens, managing second-hand smoke exposure, and maintaining a clean home environment.
- Develop an asthma action plan that includes clear instructions on what to do in the event of an asthma attack, including when to administer rescue medication and when to seek medical attention.

What to say:
- "Based on what we've discussed, we might need to adjust your inhaler or medication to better control your asthma. We'll also create an asthma action plan that you can follow at home in case of an attack."
- "It's important to keep Alex away from things that could trigger an asthma attack, like pollen or dust. Let's look at ways to improve the home environment to reduce exposure."
- "We will make sure Alex knows exactly what to do if he has trouble breathing, including when to use the inhaler and when to come to the hospital."

3. Provide Patient and Family Education
- Educate the child and family on proper inhaler techniques, emphasizing the importance of correct usage for maximum effectiveness.
- Teach the parents how to recognize early signs of

asthma exacerbation, such as increased coughing, wheezing, or shortness of breath, and how to respond promptly.
- Provide resources on asthma management, including information about triggers and preventive measures.

What to say:
- "I will show you how to use the inhaler correctly, as it's important to make sure the medication is delivered properly to help with breathing."
- "Look out for warning signs like coughing, wheezing, or trouble catching your breath. If you see these signs, give Alex his rescue inhaler right away."
- "Here's some information about asthma triggers and how to prevent them, like keeping the home free of smoke and dust. It will help you manage Alex's asthma more effectively."

4. Schedule Follow-Up Appointments and Arrange for School-Based Support

- Arrange for a follow-up appointment with a paediatric pulmonologist to further evaluate and monitor the child's asthma.
- Ensure that the child's school is aware of their condition and has a plan in place for managing asthma attacks during school hours, including keeping an inhaler at school and providing education to teachers.

What to say:

- "We'll schedule a follow-up with a paediatric pulmonologist in a few weeks to monitor Alex's progress and ensure the medications are working."
- "It's also important for the school to have an asthma action plan. I'll work with you to make sure they have the proper information to manage Alex's asthma at school."

연습 Scenario 4:
Managing Acute Confusion in an Elderly Patient

* **Time**: 10 minutes
* **Setting**: Medical Ward
* **Situation**: A 78-year-old patient with a urinary tract infection(UTI) is showing signs of acute confusion. Your task is to assess the patient, provide immediate interventions, and communicate effectively with the patient's family and healthcare team.

Example Scenario Description:

You are a registered nurse working on a medical ward. Mrs. Dorothy Carter, a 78-year-old patient, was admitted with a urinary tract infection and is now showing signs of acute confusion, including disorientation, agitation, and difficulty recognizing family members. This scenario evaluates your ability to assess and manage acute confusion(delirium) in an elderly patient while ensuring effective communication and a comprehensive care plan.

Candidate Instructions:

1. Assess the Patient's Condition

- Perform a quick assessment to confirm acute confusion:
- Use tools such as the Confusion Assessment Method(CAM).
- Assess for signs of pain, hypoxia, or dehydration.
- Check vital signs and review blood results for worsening infection.
- Look for contributing factors, such as medication side effects or sleep disturbances.

What to say:

- "Mrs. Carter, I'm here to check how you're feeling today. Can you tell me what day it is or where you are right now?"
- "I'll quickly check your vital signs to ensure there's no worsening of the infection that could be causing confusion."

2. Provide Immediate Interventions

- Ensure a calm, safe environment:
- Minimize noise and distractions.
- Use clear and simple communication.
- Reassure the patient with familiar items, such as a family photo or personal belongings.
- Manage immediate causes:
- Administer prescribed antibiotics for the UTI.

- Provide fluids to address dehydration if necessary.
- Collaborate with the doctor for further interventions if needed(e.g., oxygen for hypoxia).

What to say:
- "Mrs. Carter, let's sit somewhere quiet where you can feel more comfortable. I've brought your favourite blanket to help you feel at ease."
- "I'll make sure you're getting the right medication and fluids to help clear the infection and improve how you're feeling."

3. Communicate with the Family

- Reassure the family that acute confusion is common in older adults with infections and usually improves with treatment.
- Explain the steps being taken to address the confusion and infection.
- Encourage the family to assist with reorientation by visiting, bringing familiar items, or engaging the patient in light conversation.

What to say:
- "Acute confusion, or delirium, is not uncommon with infections like a UTI, especially in older adults. We are closely monitoring her and addressing the underlying infection, which should help her improve."

- "It would be helpful if you could visit frequently or bring some familiar items, like her favourite book or photo album, to help her feel more at ease."

4. Collaborate with the Healthcare Team

- Report the patient's symptoms to the doctor and request a review of medications or further investigations if needed.
- Work with a physiotherapist or occupational therapist to plan for mobility and fall prevention.
- Discuss discharge plans with the team, including follow-up care or support services for the patient and family.

What to say:

- "The patient is showing signs of acute confusion, which could be related to her infection or other factors. Could we review her current medications to rule out any contributors?"
- "I'd also like to involve a physiotherapist to help assess her mobility and reduce the risk of falls."

5. Document the Care Plan and Updates

- Record the patient's symptoms, interventions, and response to treatment in the patient's notes.
- Include any communication with the family and healthcare team.
- Document plans for further monitoring and discharge.

What to say(documentation):

- "Acute confusion noted: patient disoriented to time and place. Vital signs stable but shows signs of dehydration. Antibiotics and IV fluids administered as prescribed. Family informed and reorientation strategies implemented."

⑩ 위급한 상태의 환자 관리

Station Ten: Managing the deteriorating patient

* Time: 10 minutes
* Setting: Acute medical assessment Unit
* Situation: A patient with a history of COPD is experiencing acute respiratory distress.

✒ Example Example Scenario Description:

You are a registered nurse caring for Mr. Thomas Clark, a 72-year-old patient with chronic obstructive pulmonary disease(COPD), who is presenting with acute respiratory distress. Mr. Clark is exhibiting signs of increased work of breathing, laboured breathing, and a decrease in oxygen saturation. The patient's family is also visibly concerned about his condition. Your task is to perform a rapid assessment, provide appropriate interventions, and communicate effectively with the healthcare team to ensure optimal patient care.

당신은 만성 폐쇄성 폐질환(COPD)을 앓고 있는 72세 환자, 토마스 클락(Mr. Thomas Clark)을 돌보는 간호사입니다. 현재 클락 씨는 급성 호흡 곤란 증상을 보이고 있으며, 호흡 일량 증가, 호흡 곤란, 그리고 산소 포화도 감소와 같은 징후를 나타내고 있습니다. 환자의 가족 또한 그의 상태에 대해 눈에 띄게 걱정하고 있습니다. 당신의 과제는 신속한 평가를 수행하고 적절한 중재를 제공하며, 최적의 환자 치료를 보장하기 위해 의료팀과 효과적으로 소통하는 것입니다.

Candidate Instructions:

1. Perform a Rapid Assessment

- Assess the patient's respiratory status by checking vital signs, including respiratory rate, heart rate, and oxygen saturation levels.

환자의 호흡 상태를 사정하기 위해 호흡수, 심박수, 산소 포화도 등 활력 징후를 확인합니다.

- Listen to the patient's lung sounds to identify any abnormal findings, such as wheezing, crackles, or diminished breath sounds.

환자의 폐음을 청진하여 천명음, 수포음, 또는 호흡음 감소와 같은 이상 소견이 있는지 확인합니다.

- Observe the use of accessory muscles of respiration(e.g., neck muscles, intercostal retractions) and assess the patient's level of distress.

호흡 보조 근육(예: 목 근육, 갈비뼈 사이의 근육 사용)의 사용을 관찰하고 환자의 고통정도를 평가합니다.

- Evaluate the patient's ability to speak, noting any difficulty in forming sentences, which may indicate worsening respiratory failure.

> 환자의 말하는 능력을 평가하고 대화시 문장을 형성하는 데 어려움을 겪는지 확인합니다. 이는 호흡 부전이 악화되고 있음을 나타낼 수 있습니다.

What to say:
- "Mr. Clark, I'm going to check your breathing now. I need to know if you're feeling any tightness or difficulty when you breathe."
- "I'll listen to your lungs to see if we can find out what's causing your breathing issues."
- "We need to check your oxygen levels, so I'm going to place a small clip on your finger to measure it."

> "클락씨, 환자분의 호흡 상태를 지금 확인하겠습니다. 숨을 쉴 때 답답하거나 어려움이 있는지 말씀해주세요."
> "폐음을 청진하여 호흡 문제의 원인을 확인해 보겠습니다."
> "산소 포화도를 확인해야 하니, 손가락에 작은 클립을 붙여 측정하겠습니다."

2. Administer Oxygen Therapy and Prepare for Intubation

- Administer supplemental oxygen as prescribed, starting with a nasal cannula or non-rebreather mask, depending on the severity of the oxygen saturation drop.
- If the patient's condition does not improve, prepare for the possibility of intubation, ensuring the necessary

equipment is ready and the respiratory team is alerted.
- Maintain a calm and reassuring presence with the patient to help alleviate anxiety, which can exacerbate breathing difficulties.

> 산소 포화도가 떨어진 정도에 따라 비강 캐뉼라나 비재호흡 마스크를 사용하여 처방된 산소를 공급합니다. 환자의 상태가 호전되지 않으면, 기관 삽관 가능성에 대비하여 필요한 장비를 준비하고 호흡기 팀에 알립니다. 환자의 불안을 완화하기 위해 차분하고 안심을 주는 태도를 유지합니다. 불안은 호흡 곤란을 악화시킬 수 있습니다.

What to say:

- "I'm going to give you some oxygen to help you breathe easier, Mr. Clark. This should help improve your oxygen levels."
- "If your breathing doesn't get better, we may need to assist you more with breathing support. Let's see how the oxygen helps first."
- "I know this is difficult, but I'll be right here with you to support you through this."

> "클락 씨, 숨을 좀 더 쉽게 쉴 수 있도록 산소를 공급해드리겠습니다. 이 산소가 산소 수치를 개선하는 데 도움이 될 것입니다."
> "만약 숨쉬기가 나아지지 않으면, 더 많은 호흡 지원이 필요할 수도 있습니다. 우선 산소가 얼마나 도움이 되는지 지켜보겠습니다."
> "이 상황이 어렵다는 것을 알고 있습니다만, 제가 도와드릴 테니 걱정하지 마세요."

3. Monitor Vital Signs and Respiratory Status

- Continuously monitor the patient's oxygen saturation, respiratory rate, and heart rate.
- Watch for signs of worsening distress, such as

increased use of accessory muscles, cyanosis, or a significant drop in oxygen saturation.
- Keep track of any changes in the patient's condition and document these promptly.

> 환자의 산소 포화도, 호흡수, 심박수를 지속적으로 모니터링합니다. 보조 근육 사용 증가, 청색증 또는 산소 포화도 급격한 감소와 같은 악화 징후를 주의 깊게 관찰합니다. 환자의 상태에 변화가 있을 경우 이를 신속하게 기록하고 문서화합니다.

What to say:
- "I'm going to check your oxygen level again in a few minutes to make sure we're getting the right amount of oxygen to help you."
- "I'll also be checking your heart rate and breathing closely, so I can make sure we're moving in the right direction."

> "몇 분 후에 산소 포화도를 다시 확인해서 적절한 산소가 잘 공급되고 있는지 확인하겠습니다."
> "심박수와 호흡수를 면밀히 확인하여, 상태가 잘 나아지고 있는지 확인하도록 하겠습니다."

4. Notify the Physician and Collaborate on Management

- Notify the physician immediately about the patient's deteriorating condition and the need for further intervention.
- Collaborate with the healthcare team to adjust the treatment plan, which may include more aggressive

interventions, such as mechanical ventilation or administration of bronchodilators.
- Ensure that the physician is aware of any changes in the patient's condition, including respiratory status and vital signs.

> 환자의 상태가 악화되고 추가적인 처치가 필요함을 즉시 의사에게 알립니다. 의료 팀과 협력하여 치료 계획을 조정하며, 이는 기계적 환기나 기관지 확장제 투여와 같은 보다 적극적인 처치를 포함할 수 있습니다. 환자의 호흡 상태와 활력징후를 포함한 상태 변화를 의사에게 확실히 전달합니다.

What to say to the physician:
- "Dr. Lee, I have a 72-year-old patient with a history of COPD who is showing signs of acute respiratory distress. His oxygen saturation is dropping, and he's using accessory muscles to breathe. I've started oxygen therapy, but he's not improving."
- "We may need to consider more advanced interventions like intubation if his condition worsens."

> "Dr. Lee, COPD 병력이 있는 72세 환자가 급성 호흡 곤란 증상을 보이고 있습니다. 산소 포화도가 떨어지고 있으며, 호흡을 위해 보조 근육을 사용하고 있습니다. 산소 요법을 시작했지만 상태가 호전되지 않고 있습니다."
> "환자의 상태가 악화될 경우, 기도삽관과 같은 처치를 고려해야 할 수도 있습니다."

5. Document Findings, Interventions, and Communications
- Accurately document the initial assessment, including the patient's respiratory status, vital signs, and any interventions provided, such as oxygen therapy.

- Record any communications with the physician or respiratory team regarding the patient's care.
- Ensure that the documentation is clear, detailed, and timely, providing a complete record of the patient's condition and the care provided.

> 환자의 초기 평가 내용을 정확히 기록합니다. 여기에는 환자의 호흡 상태, 활력 징후, 산소 요법과 같은 처치가 포함됩니다. 환자의 치료와 관련하여 의사나 호흡 치료 팀과 나눈 모든 의사소통 내용을 기록합니다. 문서는 명확하고 상세하며 시기적절해야 하며, 환자의 상태와 제공된 치료에 대한 기록을 제공합니다.

What to say:
- "I'm going to note everything we've done so far in your chart to ensure we have a full record of your care today. This will help keep track of your progress."

> "환자분, 오늘 치료 과정을 완전하게 남기기 위해 지금까지 했던 모든 것을 차트에 기록하겠습니다. 이것은 당신의 상태가 어떻게 나아지고 있는지 추적하는 데 도움이 될 것입니다."

연습 Scenario 1:
Acute Gastrointestinal Bleed

* Time: 10 minutes
* Setting: Emergency Department
* Situation: A patient presents with signs of gastrointestinal bleeding, including melena, hypotension, and tachycardia.

Example Scenario Description:

Mr. Brian Hudson, a 55-year-old male, is admitted to the emergency department with complaints of black, tarry stools(melena), dizziness, and a rapid heart rate. He has a history of peptic ulcer disease and is at risk for an acute gastrointestinal bleed. Immediate intervention is necessary to prevent shock and further complications.

Candidate Instructions:

1. Perform a Rapid Assessment of Vital Signs and Symptoms

- Assess the patient's vital signs, particularly blood pressure and heart rate, which may indicate hemodynamic instability due to blood loss.
- Obtain a focused history of symptoms, including the onset of melena, associated pain, and any history of GI issues(e.g., ulcers or recent anticoagulant use).

What to say:

- "Mr. Hudson, I need to check your blood pressure and heart rate to see how you're doing right now. Let me know if you feel lightheaded or faint."
- "We'll also ask about your symptoms, including any stomach pain or recent history of ulcers."

2. Administer IV Fluids and Prepare for Possible Blood Transfusion

- Start intravenous fluid resuscitation with normal saline or lactated Ringer's to stabilize blood pressure.
- Prepare for a potential blood transfusion if the patient shows signs of significant blood loss.

What to say:

- "I'm going to start an IV and give you fluids to help with your blood pressure. This should make you feel a little better."

> "We may need to give you some blood if the bleeding doesn't stop, but we'll see how things go."

3. Monitor Vital Signs and Symptoms

> Monitor for any signs of shock, such as a significant drop in blood pressure or an increase in heart rate.
> Keep track of the patient's urine output to assess renal perfusion and signs of hypoperfusion.

What to say:
> "I'll keep monitoring your blood pressure and heart rate closely, Mr. Hudson. Let me know if you feel any different."

4. Notify the Physician and Coordinate for Endoscopic Evaluation

> Notify the physician immediately and prepare for endoscopy to locate the source of bleeding.
> Alert the gastroenterology team to assist with an urgent assessment and management of the GI bleed.

What to say to the physician:
> "Dr. Garcia, Mr. Hudson is showing signs of gastrointestinal bleeding with melena and hypotension. He needs immediate fluid resuscitation and endoscopic evaluation."

5. Document Findings and Actions

↠ Record all vital signs, symptoms, interventions(IV fluids, transfusions), and communications with the physician in the patient's chart.

What to say:

↠ "I'll document everything so that all the steps we've taken are clearly recorded and available

연습 Scenario 2:
Atrial Fibrillation with Rapid Ventricular Response(RVR)

* Time: 10 minutes
* Setting: Emergency Department
* Situation: A patient with atrial fibrillation is experiencing rapid ventricular response(RVR) and significant symptoms.

Example Scenario Description:

Ms. Emily Green, a 72-year-old female with a known history of atrial fibrillation(AF), presents to the emergency department with complaints of palpitations, dizziness, and shortness of breath. Her heart rate is elevated at 150 beats per minute, and she is in atrial fibrillation with rapid ventricular response(RVR). The patient reports feeling weak and anxious due to the heart rate and associated symptoms. Immediate management is required to control the rate and prevent complications such as thromboembolism.

✒ Candidate Instructions:

1. Perform a Rapid Assessment and Monitoring

- Assess the patient's vital signs, particularly heart rate, blood pressure, oxygen saturation, and respiratory status.
- Ask the patient about any chest pain, dizziness, or light-headedness, as these can be signs of hemodynamic instability.
- Obtain a 12-lead ECG to confirm the presence of atrial fibrillation and rapid ventricular response.

What to say:

- "Ms. Green, I'm going to check your vital signs, including your heart rate, and make sure you're comfortable. I'll also perform an ECG to see how your heart is beating."
- "Can you tell me if you feel any chest pain or light-headedness? I want to make sure we take care of everything."

2. Administer Medications to Control Heart Rate

- Administer medications as ordered to control the heart rate, such as beta-blockers(e.g., metoprolol) or calcium channel blockers(e.g., diltiazem).
- Consider anticoagulation therapy if the patient's atrial fibrillation is new or has lasted for more than 48 hours, to prevent clot formation and stroke.

What to say:

- "We're going to give you some medication to help slow down your heart rate and make you feel more comfortable. This will help manage the rapid rhythm."
- "We may also give you some blood thinners to prevent clots from forming because atrial fibrillation can increase the risk of stroke."

3. Continuous Monitoring and Patient Observation

- Continuously monitor the patient's heart rate and rhythm via ECG to assess the effectiveness of treatment.
- Monitor blood pressure and oxygen saturation to assess for any signs of hypoperfusion or respiratory distress.
- Observe for any signs of stroke or hemodynamic instability, such as altered mental status or significant hypotension.

What to say:

- "I'm going to keep monitoring your heart rate closely and make sure your blood pressure stays stable. If you feel any worsening symptoms, let me know immediately."

4. Notify the Physician and Discuss Further Management

- Contact the physician or cardiologist to update them on the patient's condition, discuss the treatment plan, and

obtain further orders.
- Discuss potential interventions, such as electrical cardioversion or additional medications(e.g., digoxin or amiodarone), if the rate is not well controlled.

What to say to the physician:
- "Dr. Lee, Ms. Green is in atrial fibrillation with rapid ventricular response at 150 bpm. We've started metoprolol and are monitoring her closely. Should we consider further interventions or cardioversion?"

5. Document the Care Provided
- Record all vital signs, ECG findings, medications administered, and patient responses to treatment in the patient's chart.
- Document communications with the physician and any changes in the patient's condition.

What to say:
- "I'm going to document everything we've done, including the medications and monitoring so that we have a complete record of your care."

연습 Scenario 3:
Fall in a Hospitalized Patient with Signs of Deterioration

* **Time**: 10 minutes
* **Setting**: Medical Ward
* **Situation**: A patient experienced a fall and is now showing signs of deterioration, including confusion, low blood pressure, and increased heart rate.

Example Scenario Description:

Mr. James Anderson, a 68-year-old patient admitted for pneumonia, was found on the floor by a staff member after attempting to walk to the bathroom unassisted. The patient is now presenting with concerning symptoms, including confusion, a heart rate of 110 bpm, a blood pressure of 88/54 mmHg, and pallor. He denies hitting his head but complains of hip pain. You are the nurse assigned to assess his condition, provide immediate interventions, and escalate care as needed.

Candidate Instructions:

1. Assess the Patient's Condition

- Perform a rapid head-to-toe assessment, focusing on injuries from the fall and any signs of hemodynamic instability, such as hypotension or tachycardia.
- Check vital signs, including blood pressure, heart rate, respiratory rate, oxygen saturation, and temperature.
- Assess the level of consciousness and orientation, noting any confusion or changes in mental status.
- Ask the patient about pain, particularly in the hip, and whether they hit their head or lost consciousness.

What to say:

- "Mr. Anderson, I'm going to check you over thoroughly to make sure you're okay. Let me know if you feel any pain or discomfort while I examine you."
- "Can you tell me if you're feeling dizzy or confused? Did you hit your head or lose consciousness when you fell?"

2. Provide Immediate Care

- If the patient is unable to get up safely, call for assistance to transfer the patient to bed or a safe position using proper techniques.
- Manage any visible injuries, such as applying ice to bruises or providing pain relief as appropriate.
- Administer oxygen if oxygen saturation is below normal.

What to say:

- "We're going to get you back to bed safely. Please don't move on your own; let us assist you."
- "Let's apply an ice pack to your hip to help with the swelling, and I'll give you some pain relief shortly."

3. Escalate Care for Signs of Deterioration

- Notify the physician immediately about the patient's symptoms, including low blood pressure, tachycardia, and confusion.
- Prepare for diagnostic imaging, such as X-rays or CT scans, to assess for fractures or internal injuries.
- Monitor for potential complications, such as internal bleeding or head trauma, even if the patient denies hitting their head.

What to say to the physician:

- "Dr. Lee, Mr. Anderson experienced a fall and is now showing signs of deterioration. His blood pressure is 88/54 mmHg, heart rate is 110 bpm, and he's confused. He's also complaining of hip pain. Would you like to order imaging or labs to rule out internal injuries?"

What to say to the patient:

- "Mr. Anderson, I've noticed your blood pressure is a little low, and I'm going to call the doctor to make sure we address this quickly."

↠ "We'll run some tests to ensure there are no hidden injuries or other concerns from the fall."

4. Monitor the Patient Closely

↠ Continuously monitor the patient's vital signs, level of consciousness, and pain level to identify any further deterioration.
↠ Watch for additional symptoms, such as increased confusion, cyanosis, or a further drop in blood pressure.

What to say:

↠ "I'm going to monitor your blood pressure, heart rate, and oxygen levels closely to make sure you're stable. If you feel worse or notice any new symptoms, let me know immediately."

5. Implement Fall Prevention Strategies

↠ Collaborate with the healthcare team to implement fall prevention measures, such as using a bed alarm, ensuring the call bell is within reach, and assisting the patient with all mobility needs.
↠ Educate the patient on the importance of asking for help before attempting to get out of bed.

What to say:

↣ "To keep you safe, we're going to put some additional measures in place, like keeping the bed alarm on and making sure someone assists you every time you get up."

↣ "Please use the call bell before moving. We're here to help, and your safety is our priority."

6. Document the Event and Interventions

↣ Record the details of the fall, including the time, location, and any symptoms or injuries observed.

↣ Document vital signs, interventions provided, and communication with the physician.

What to say:

↣ "I'm going to document everything we've done so far, including your vital signs, the care we provided, and the doctor's instructions. This will help ensure we track your progress and keep you safe."

연습 Scenario 4:
Deteriorating Post-Angioplasty Patient

* Time: 10 minutes
* Setting: Post-Procedure Recovery Unit
* Situation: A patient who has undergone angioplasty with stent placement is exhibiting signs of deterioration, including hypotension, chest pain, and shortness of breath. Immediate intervention is required to stabilize the patient and prevent further complications.

Example Scenario Description:

Mr. Robert Davis, a 68-year-old male, recently underwent coronary angioplasty with stent placement for a coronary artery blockage. His procedure was initially uncomplicated, but 2 hours post-procedure, he began to exhibit signs of deterioration. He is complaining of sudden chest pain, his blood pressure has dropped to 85/50 mmHg, and his oxygen saturation is decreasing to 88% on room air. His heart rate is elevated at 110 bpm, and he appears anxious and restless. You are tasked with assessing his condition, providing immediate interventions, and communicating effectively with the healthcare team to address the developing situation.

Candidate Instructions:

1. Rapid Assessment and Monitoring

- Assess the patient's vital signs, particularly blood pressure, heart rate, respiratory rate, and oxygen saturation.
- Perform an ECG to assess the rhythm and check for signs of myocardial ischemia or arrhythmia.
- Assess for signs of worsening chest pain, shortness of breath, or sweating, which may indicate re-occlusion of the stented artery or myocardial infarction.

What to say:

- "Mr. Davis, I'm going to check your vital signs right now. Are you feeling more pain or discomfort? Let me know if your chest pain gets worse."
- "I'm also going to perform an ECG to monitor your heart's rhythm and see if there's anything that needs urgent attention."

2. Administer Oxygen and Ensure IV Access

- Administer supplemental oxygen via a nasal cannula or non-rebreather mask to improve oxygen saturation.

- Ensure that the IV line is patent for administering any necessary medications, such as fluids, vasopressors, or pain relief.
- Start IV fluids to help stabilize the patient's blood pressure.

What to say:
- "I'm going to give you some oxygen to help you breathe easier. This will help increase your oxygen levels and ease your discomfort."
- "We'll also start an IV line for fluids to help support your blood pressure and improve your circulation."

3. Assess the Stent Insertion Site for Complications

- Reassess the catheter insertion site for signs of bleeding, hematoma, or arterial occlusion.
- Apply pressure if there's any sign of bleeding and alert the physician if any complications are identified at the access site.
- If there are concerns about arterial occlusion or significant bleeding, prepare for further interventions such as a vascular consult or additional diagnostic imaging.

What to say:
- "I'll check the area where the catheter was inserted to ensure there's no bleeding or swelling. It's important we make sure the insertion site is stable."

- "If there's any bleeding, we may need to apply more pressure to help control it. Let me know if you feel any new pain or tenderness in that area."

4. Administer Medications to Address the Deterioration

- Administer pain relief as prescribed to manage the patient's chest pain.
- Administer medications such as nitro-glycerine(if prescribed) to alleviate chest pain if ischemia is suspected.
- Notify the physician to discuss the potential need for more aggressive interventions such as thrombolytics or urgent revascularization.

What to say:

- "We're going to give you some medication to help with your chest pain and ease your discomfort. This should help improve your symptoms."
- "I'm also going to check in with the doctor to see if we need to take further steps, like using medications to dissolve any potential clot or discussing more advanced treatments."

5. Continuous Monitoring and Observation

- Continuously monitor the patient's heart rate, blood pressure, oxygen saturation, and ECG for any signs of further deterioration or myocardial ischemia.

- Observe for any signs of shock or worsening ischemia, such as increasing tachycardia, decreasing urine output, or altered mental status.
- Be prepared to escalate care if the patient's condition continues to worsen.

What to say:
- "I'm going to keep a close eye on your heart rate, blood pressure, and oxygen levels. If anything changes, we'll act quickly to make sure we manage this properly."
- "Let me know immediately if you feel any worsening pain or discomfort."

6. Notify the Physician and Discuss Immediate Interventions

- Immediately contact the physician or cardiologist to update them on the patient's deteriorating condition and discuss possible interventions.
- Discuss the potential need for further diagnostic tests, such as a repeat angiogram or urgent coronary intervention.
- If the patient's symptoms worsen, prepare for the potential need for additional treatments, including the use of thrombolytics or transfer to a higher level of care(e.g., intensive care unit).

What to say to the physician:

➤ "Dr. Lee, Mr. Davis is showing signs of deterioration. He is experiencing chest pain, hypotension(85/50 mmHg), and decreased oxygen saturation(88%). We've initiated oxygen and IV fluids, but his condition is not improving. Should we consider further interventions, such as a repeat angiogram or thrombolytics?"

7. Document the Care Provided and Communication

➤ Accurately document the patient's vital signs, symptoms, interventions provided, and responses to treatment.
➤ Record any communications with the healthcare team and any changes in the patient's condition.
➤ Ensure that the documentation reflects all steps taken to manage the deteriorating situation and communicate with the physician.

What to say:

➤ "I'll document everything we've done today, including the changes in your condition, the medications we've administered, and the actions we've taken to manage your care."

OSCE 준비
꿀팁!

OSCE 준비 관련 도서

1. Smeltzer, S. C., Bare, B., Hinkle, J., & Cheever, K. H.(2020). Brunner and Suddarth's Textbook of Medical-Surgical Nursing(15th ed.).
   - 임상적 판단과 기술 연습을 위한 기본 교재.

2. Berman, A., Snyder, S., & Frandsen, G.(2020). Kozier and Erb's Fundamentals of Nursing(11th ed.).
   - 간호 기본 원칙과 실습 방법.

3. Jarvis, C.(2019). Physical Examination and Health Assessment(8th ed.).
   - 신체 검진 및 건강 평가 스킬.

4. OSCE and Clinical Skills Handbook
   Author: Katrina F. Hurley, Peter Green and Rose P. Mengual
   - 이 책은 의학 교육 중 학생들이 습득해야 할 기본적인 병력 청취 및 신체 검사 기술을 요약하여 Q&A 형식으로 제시합니다. 이를 통해 개인 학습과 그룹 학습 모두를 효율적으로 지원할 수 있도록 구성되었습니다.

5. Passing Your Advanced Nursing OSCE
A Guide to Success in Advanced Clinical Skills Assessment(MasterPass Series)
Author: Ward, Helen, Barratt, Julian, Navreet Paul

- 이 책은 고급 간호 실습 능력을 평가하는 실습 시험과 비의료 처방 평가를 준비하는 학생들을 위한 실용적인 참고서입니다. OSCE 시나리오에서 잘 수행할 수 있도록 단계별 지침을 제공하며, OSCE 준비와 채점에 대한 가이드를 제공합니다.

6. Nursing objective structured clinical examination(OSCE)
Author: Heba Abdel Mowla

- 이 책은 간호학교에서 수행되는 성과 기반 시험을 위한 OSCE(객관적 구조화 임상 시험) 사례 개발 및 검토에 대한 지침을 제공합니다. 또한, OSCE 사례 개발의 8단계 과정을 설명하며, 이를 통해 간호 학생들의 능력을 공정하고 유효하게 평가할 수 있도록 돕는 것을 목표로 합니다.

7. Nursing OSCEs; A Complete Guide to Exam Success
Author: Catherine Cabellero(Edited by), Fiona Creed(Edited by), Clare Gochmanski, Jane Lovegrove(Edited by)

- 학생 친화적이고 실용적인 복습 가이드로, 가장 일반적으로 평가되는 10가지 기술에 대한 단계별 설명과 예시 채점표, 전형적인 시험관 질문 및 제안된 답변을 제공합니다. 70개 이상의 삽화와 4개의 동영상을 통해 성공적인 시험 준비를 돕는 책입니다.

OSCE 준비를 위한 웹사이트

1

New Zealand Nursing Council.
- 공식 홈페이지: https://www.nursingcouncil.org.nz
- 뉴질랜드 간호사의 등록기준, 윤리및 실무 지침 제공

2

https://www.hqsc.govt.nz/our-work/leadership-and-capability/kaiawhina-workforce/health-literacy-equity-cultural-safety-and-competence/

- 뉴질랜드의 다문화 환경에서 환자를 안전하게 간호하는 방법을 제시

3

Ministry of Health New Zealand
- 공식 홈페이지: https://www.health.govt.nz
- 뉴질랜드의 보건 정책 및 문화적 안전성 정보.

4

Te Pou o te Whakaaro Nui(Mental Health Support)

- 공식 홈페이지: https://www.tepou.co.nz
- 정신건강 및 장애 지원 관련 자원.

ACC(Accident Compensation Corporation)

- 공식 홈페이지: https://www.acc.co.nz
- 환자의 재활 및 보상 관련 정보.

Geeky Medics

- 웹사이트: https://geekymedics.com
- OSCE 관련 시뮬레이션 동영상, 팁, 평가 시트 제공.

OSCEstop

- 웹사이트: https://oscestop.com
- OSCE 준비를 위한 무료 리소스 및 평가 체크리스트.

Nursing Times

- 웹사이트: https://www.nursingtimes.net
- 최신 간호 뉴스와 연구 자료.

OSCE 준비 앱 및 온라인 자료

1

Medscape App
- 간호 및 의료 정보를 신속히 검색할 수 있는 앱.
- 다운로드: https://www.medscape.com

2

Quizlet
- OSCE 키워드와 주요 개념 암기를 위한 플래시카드 도구.
- 링크: https://quizlet.com

3

Elsevier Clinical Skills
- 임상 기술 연습을 위한 온라인 자료.
- 링크: https://clinicalskills.net

4

Nursing OSCE App
- OSCE 준비를 위한 모바일 애플리케이션(iOS/Android).

5

그외 엄청난 Youtube 자료들

이 자료와 리소스들은 뉴질랜드 OSCE 준비뿐만 아니라 실무에서 지속적으로 활용할 수 있는 유용한 참고 자료가 될 것입니다. 이를 통해 시험뿐만 아니라 실무에서도 간호사로서의 자신감을 가질 수 있도록 돕는 것이 목표입니다.

마무리 하며

뉴질랜드 간호사가 되기 위한 마지막 관문, OSCE 준비의 의미

뉴질랜드 간호사가 되기 위해 거쳐야 하는 OSCE(객관적 구조화된 임상 시험)는 단순한 시험 이상의 의미를 갖습니다. 이는 간호사로서의 임상 능력, 문제 해결력, 그리고 환자 중심의 접근 방식을 실무에서 얼마나 효과적으로 적용할 수 있는지를 검증하는 중요한 과정입니다.

OSCE는 간호사의 역할과 책임, 윤리적 실천, 그리고 문화적 안전성을 평가하며, 실제 임상 환경에서 발생할 수 있는 다양한 상황을 기반으로 구성됩니다.

이 책은 뉴질랜드 OSCE 준비를 돕기 위해 철저히 설계되었습니다.

각 스테이션별 목표와 평가 기준, 실전 팁, 그리고 실제 시나리오 예시를 통해 시험에서 요구되는 핵심 역량을 명확히 이해하고 연습할 수 있도록 도울 것입니다. 무엇보다, 이 과정은 단지 시험을 통과하기 위한 준비가 아니라, 뉴질랜드 간호사로서 환자와 가족에게 최상의 간호를 제공할 수 있는 자신감을 쌓는 과정이기도 합니다.

OSCE 준비: 성장과 배움의 과정

OSCE 준비 과정은 단순히 기술 습득에 그치지 않고, 간호사의 전반적인 성장과 전문성을 강화하는 데 기여합니다.

1. 환자 중심의 간호

뉴질랜드 간호는 환자의 목소리를 경청하고, 그들의 필요를 존중하며, 개인화된 간호를 계획하는 데 초점을 둡니다. OSCE 준비를 통해 환자 중심의 접근법을 실질적으로 익힐 수 있습니다.

2. 임상적 자신감

실제 상황과 유사한 시뮬레이션 연습은 시험뿐만 아니라 실무에서도 자신감을 가질 수 있는 기반을 제공합니다. 이는 다양한 임상 환경에서 문제를 신속히 파악하고, 적절한 해결책을 제시할 수 있는 능력을 길러줍니다.

3. 시간 관리와 명확한 소통

제한된 시간 내에 효율적으로 과제를 수행하고, 간결하면서도 정확한 의사소통과 문서화를 연습한 경험은 실무에서도 큰 자산이 됩니다.

4. 문화적 안전성의 이해

뉴질랜드는 다문화 사회로, 간호사는 다양한 배경을 가진 환자와 가족을 배려하며 간호를 제공해야 합니다. OSCE 준비는 이러한 문화적 안전성을 실무에 반영할 수 있는 중요한 기회를 제공합니다.

뉴질랜드 간호사의 길로 나아가기

OSCE는 간호사로서의 전문성과 실력을 입증할 수 있는 중요한 과정입니다. 이를 통과하는 것은 단지 시험 합격을 의미하는 것이 아니라, 뉴질랜드 의료 체계에서 간호사로서 환자와 가족의 삶에 긍정적인 영향을 미칠 준비가 되었음을 나타냅니다. 또한 OSCE를 준비하며 습득한 지식과 기술은 시험 이후의 실무에서도 계속 활용되며, 환자의 건강과 웰빙을 증진시키는 데 기여할 것입니다.

이 책은 여러분이 OSCE를 자신감 있게 준비하고 성공적으로 통과할 수 있도록 돕는 동반자 역할을 할 것입니다. 시험 준비 과정에서 배우고 익힌 모든 것이 단지 합격을 넘어, 뉴질랜드의 간호사로서 훌륭한 첫걸음을 내딛는 데 중요한 밑거름이 되기를 바랍니다.

뉴질랜드 간호사가 되기 위해 노력해 온 모든분들에게 진심으로 응원의 메시지를 보냅니다. 이제 여러분의 다음 여정을 시작할 시간입니다.

성공적인 간호사로서의 앞날에 축복이 가득하길 기원합니다!

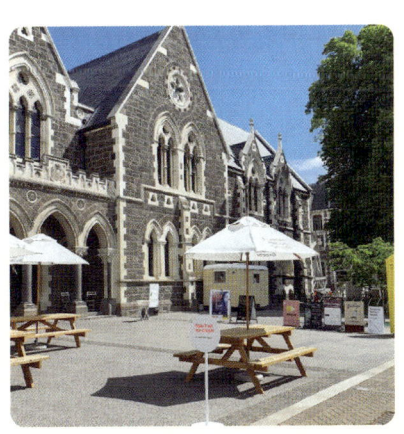

❖ 포널스 참고문헌

장수향. (2018). 뉴질랜드 간호사 되기. 포널스.

김미연. (2019). 국제간호사 길라잡이. 포널스.

손정화. (2020). 국제간호사 호주편. 포널스.

송원경. (2021). 국제간호사 두바이편. 포널스.

정해빛나. (2021). 국제간호사 미국편. 포널스.

김소미. (2022). 국제간호사 사우디, 조지아편. 포널스.

간호사적응연구소. (2023). 병원적응 의학용어. 포널스.

간호사적응연구소. (2023). 국제간호사 병원영어 Vol1 - 말하기 편. 포널스.

간호사적응연구소. (2023). 국제간호사 병원영어 Vol2 - 간호상황 편. 포널스.

백소연. (2024). 미국간호사 밥줄영어 vol 1권. 포널스.

백소연. (2024). 미국간호사 밥줄영어 vol 2권. 포널스.

간호사타임즈. (2024). 태어난 김에 국제간호사. 포널스.

윤보혜. (2024). 국제간호사 호주(탈임상)편. 포널스.

이지원. (2024). 미국 부자 간호사 가난한 간호사. 포널스.

강은진. (2025). 선넘는 간호사 - 호주간호사로 선넘다. 포널스.

간호사연구소. (2025). 간호알고리즘 PRO-A1 호흡기내과. 포널스.

간호사연구소. (2025). 간호알고리즘 PRO-A2 심장내과. 포널스.

간호사연구소. (2025). 간호알고리즘 PRO-A3 혈액종양내과. 포널스.

간호사연구소. (2025). 간호알고리즘 PRO-A4 소화기내과/간담췌내과. 포널스.

간호사연구소. (2025). 간호알고리즘 PRO-A5 신장내과. 포널스.

간호사연구소. (2025). 간호알고리즘 PRO-A6 일반외과/정형외과. 포널스.

간호사연구소. (2025). 간호알고리즘 PRO-A7 신경외과. 포널스.